SIRT "FOOD" DIET

An easy guide with delicious and healthy recipes to stay fit and lose weight. Activate your **skinny gene** for fat burning!

By Vilma J. Hernandez.

Table of Contents

Introduction

The basis of the sirtuin diet can be explained in simple terms or complex ways. It is essential to understand how and why it works, however, to appreciate the value of what you are doing. It is also necessary to know why these sirtuin rich foods help you maintain fidelity to your diet plan. Otherwise, you may throw something in your meal with less nutrition that would defeat the purpose of planning for one rich in sirtuins. Most importantly, this is not a dietary fad, and as you will see, there is much wisdom in how humans have used natural foods even for medicinal purposes, over thousands of years.

To understand how the Sirtfood diet works and why these particular foods are necessary, we will look at their role in the human body.

Sirtuin activity was first researched in yeast, where a mutation caused an extension in the yeast's lifespan. Sirtuins were also shown to slow aging in laboratory mice, fruit flies, and nematodes. As Sirtuins' research proved to transfer to mammals, they were examined for their use in diet and slowing the aging process. The sirtuins in humans are different in typing, but they essentially work in the same ways and reasons.

There are seven "members" that make up the sirtuin family. It is believed that sirtuins play a significant role in regulating certain functions of cells, including proliferation (reproduction and growth of cells), apoptosis (death of cells). They promote survival and resist stress to increase longevity.

They are also seen to block neurodegeneration (loss of function of the brain's nerve cells). They conduct their housekeeping functions by cleaning out toxic proteins and supporting the brain's ability to change and adapt to different conditions or recuperate (i.e., brain plasticity). As part of this, they also help reduce chronic inflammation and reduce something called oxidative stress. Oxidative stress is when there are too many cell-damaging free radicals circulating in the body, and the body cannot catch up by combating them with anti-oxidants. These factors are related to age-related illness and weight, which again brings us back to how they work.

You will see labels in Sirtuins that start with "SIR," representing "Silence Information Regulator" genes. They do precisely that, silence or regulate, as part of their functions. The seven sirtuins humans work with are SIRT1, SIRT2, SIRT3, SIRT4, SIRT 5, SIRT6, and SIRT7. Each of these types is responsible for different areas of protecting cells. They work by either stimulating or turning on certain gene expressions or reducing and turning off other gene expressions. It essentially means that they can influence genes to do more or less of something, most of which they are already programmed to do.

Through enzyme reactions, each of the SIRT types affects different cells responsible for the metabolic processes that help maintain life. It is also related to what organs and functions they will act.

For example, SIRT6 causes the expression of the genes in humans that affect skeletal muscle, fat tissue, brain, and heart. SIRT 3 would induce an expression of genes that affect the kidneys, liver, brain, and heart.

If we tie these concepts together, you can see that the Sirtuin proteins can change the expression of genes, and in the case of the Sirtfood Diet, we care about how sirtuins can turn off those genes that are responsible for speeding up aging and for weight management.

The other aspect to this conversation of sirtuins is the function and the power of calorie restriction on the human body. Calorie restriction is merely eating fewer calories. It, coupled with exercise and reducing stress, is usually a combination of weight loss. Calorie restriction has also proven across much research in animals and humans to increase one's lifespan.

We can look further at the role of sirtuins with calorie restriction and using the SIRT3 protein, which has a role in metabolism and aging. Amongst all of the effects of the protein on gene expression (such as preventing cells from dying, reducing tumors from growing, etc.), we want to understand the impact of SIRT3 on weight for this book.

As we stated earlier, the SIRT3 has high expression in those metabolically active tissues, and its ability to express itself increases with caloric restriction, fasting, and exercise. On the contrary, it will express itself less when the body has high fat, high-calorie-riddled diet.

The last few highlights of sirtuins are their role in regulating telomeres and reducing inflammation, which also helps prevent disease and aging.

Telomeres are sequences of proteins at the ends of chromosomes. When cells divide, these get shorter. As we age, they get shorter, and other stressors to the body also will contribute to this. Maintaining these longer telomeres is the key to slower aging. Also, proper diet, along with exercise and other variables, can lengthen telomeres. SIRT6 is one of the sirtuins that, if activated, can help with DNA damage, inflammation, and oxidative stress. SIRT1 also helps with inflammatory response cycles that are related to many age-related diseases.

Calories restriction, as we mentioned earlier, can extend life to some degree. Since this and fasting are a stressor, these factors will stimulate the SIRT3 proteins to kick in and protect the body from the stressors and excess free radicals. Again, the telomere length is affected as well.

To sum up, all of this information also shows that, contrary to some people's beliefs, genetics, such as "it is what it is" or "it is my fate because Uncle Joe has something..." through our own lifestyle choices. To what we are exposed to, we can influence action and changes in our genes. It is quite an empowering thought, yet another reason you should be excited to have a science-based diet such as the Sirtfood diet is available to you.

Having laid this all out before you, you should be able to appreciate how and why these miraculous compounds work in your favor to keep you youthful, healthy, and lean. If they are working hard for you, don't you feel that you should do something too? Well, you can, and that is what the rest of this book will do for you by providing all the SIRT-recipes.

The Advantages Of The Sirt Diet

Sirtuins are a group of 7 proteins that maintain cell metabolism and homeostasis at optimal levels. Three of these proteins are found in the mitochondria, the cytoplasm, and another three are located in the nucleus. Sirtuins maintain the cell's health and ensure that all processes going on within the cell are properly happening. Sirtuins can, however, not be effective without the presence of NAD+ (nicotinamide adenine dinucleotide). NAD+ is a coenzyme that is present in all cells that are living in nature. NAD+ ensures that Sirtuins function optimally and can regulate cells.

Homeostasis within the cell maintains all the numerous functions of the cell at stability, which ensures balance. It may also involve the maintenance of PH and the saturate concentration levels of the cytoplasm, which is the most significant cell component in terms of volume. All these are aspects of the cell that must stay constant for optimal cell health. Sirtuins perform several functions, among them being the ability to deacetylase proteins called histones. Acetyls are proteins with a physical form of Histones are proteins that contain a condensed form of DNA called chromatins, which prevent the proteins from performing their functions in this acetyl.

The deacetylation frees the proteins for their respective functions, given that proteins are the building blocks for the body. Proteins are proverbially referred to as bodybuilding foods. Without Sirtuins, therefore, the bodybuilding foods would fail to build our bodies as they are the critical components for freeing the protein molecules in our cells for their functions.

The Miracle of the Blue Areas

The other evidence for the power of Sirtfoods comes from the 'blue zones.' The blue zones are small regions in the world where people miraculously live longer than everywhere else.

Perhaps most startlingly, you don't just see people live longer in blue zones; you still see them retain energy, vigor, and overall health even in their advanced years. Many of us have a fear of becoming decrepit, immobile, and overall miserable as we age.

Furthermore, we envision this as starting to occur in our forties and fifties while becoming a fixed reality in our sixties, seventies, and eighties. Yet in the blue zones, people live past 100 surprisingly regularly but can walk, work and exercise just as well as those in the younger years. Likewise, they remain mentally capable and don't suffer the cognitive deficits we typically associate with old age.

The blue zones include several areas of the Mediterranean, Japan, Italy, and Costa Rica. What do these regions all have in common? They all eat a diet high in Sirt foods. The Mediterranean is famous for its healthy diet involving copious amounts of fish and olive oil. The Japanese savor matcha green tea, while the Costa Ricans traditionally indulge in cocoa, coffee, and more.

The beauty of the Sirt food diet isn't trying to make your eating habits artificial and awkward. It is merely copying the healthiest practices that already exist around the world.

Sirt Diet and Muscle Mass

There is a family of genes that function as guardians of our muscle in the body. Also, when under stress, avoid its breakdown, it is known as the sirtuins. SIRT is a potent Muscle Breakdown Inhibitor. As long as SIRT is activated, even when we are fasting, muscle breakdown is prevented, and we continue to burn fat for fuel.

SIRT's benefits aren't ending with preserving muscle mass. The sirtuins work to increase our skeletal muscle mass. We need to explore into the exciting world of stem cells and illustrate how that process functions. Our muscle comprises a particular type of stem cell called a satellite cell that regulates its development and regeneration. Satellite cells sit there quietly most of the time, but they are activated when a muscle gets damaged or stressed. By things like weight training, this is how our muscles grow stronger. SIRT is essential for activating satellite cells, and without its activity, muscles are significantly smaller because they no longer have the capacity to develop or regenerate properly. However, by increasing SIRT activity, we boost our satellite cells, encouraging muscle growth and recovery.

Sirt Diet and Goodness

There was one aspect we couldn't get our minds around in our pilot study: the people didn't get hungry given a drop-in calorie. In reality, several people struggled to consume all of the food that was offered. One of the significant advantages of the Sirtfood Diet is that we can achieve significant benefits without the need for a long-term calorie restriction. The very first week of diet is the process of hyper-success, where we pair mild fasting with an excess of strong Sirtfoods for a double blow to weight. So, we predicted sure signs of hunger here, as with all of the fasting regimens. But we've had virtually zero!

We found the answer as we trawled through analysis. It's all thanks to the body's primary appetite-regulating hormone, leptin, called the "satiety hormone." As we feed, leptin decreases, signaling the hypothalamus inhibiting desire to a part of the brain. Conversely, leptin signaling to the mind declines as we fly, which makes us feel thirsty.

Leptin is so effective in controlling appetite that early expectations where it could be treated as a "magic bullet" for combating obesity. But that vision was broken because the metabolic disorder found in obesity causes leptin to avoid correctly functioning. Through obesity, the volume of leptin that can reach the brain is not only decreased. But the hypothalamus also becomes desensitized to its behavior. It is regarded as leptin resistance: there is leptin, but it doesn't work correctly anymore. Therefore, for many overweight individuals, the brain continues to think they are underfed even though they consume plenty, which triggers them to seek calories.

The consequence of this is that while the amount of leptin in the blood is necessary to control appetite, how much of it enters the brain and can affect the hypothalamus is far more relevant. It is here that the Sirtfoods shine.

New evidence indicates that the nutrients present in Sirtfoods have unique advantages in overcoming leptin resistance. By increasing leptin delivery to the brain and through the hypothalamus ' response to leptin behavior.

Going back to our original question on why don't the Sirtfood Diet make people feel hungry? Given a decrease in blood leptin rates during the mild quick, which would usually raise motivation, incorporating Sirtfoods into the diet makes leptin signals more productive, leading to better appetite control. Sirtfoods also have powerful effects on our taste centers, meaning we get a lot more pleasure and satisfaction from our food. Therefore, don't fall into the overeating trap to feel happy. Sirtuins are expected to be a brand-new concept for even the most committed dietitians. But hitting the sirtuins, our metabolism's master regulators, is the foundation of any effective diet for weight loss. Tragically, the very existence of our modern society, with abundant food and sedentary lifestyles, creates a perfect storm to shut down our sirtuin operation, and we see all around us the effects of this.

The good thing is that we know what sirtuins are, how fat accumulation is managed, and how fat burning is encouraged, and most significantly, how to turn them on. And with this revolutionary breakthrough, the key to successful and lasting weight loss is now yours to bear.

Maintaining The Sirtfood Diet

After the successful beginning of the Sirtfood diet, there is more work to do. You need to ensure that the morale and momentum you had at the beginning of the diet are maintained to complete the diet. In this regard, the tips given have been tested and confirmed to help people manage the motivation and morale for completing the Sirtfood diet.

Check-In with Your Set Goals

You have understood the importance of setting goals at the inception of the Sirtfood diet. These goals need to attainable and realistic to allow for adherence to it. However, these realistic goals that you have set need to be checked continuously during the diet. Continually checking in with your set goals reminds you of the reason for starting the diet in the first place. It brings up the image of the future you had in mind at the beginning of the Sirtfood diet. By checking your set target during the diet course, the primary source of motivation and inspiration for the diet is revived, thus giving you enough will continue with the Sirtfood diet no matter the difficulties encountered. Apart from reviving the motivation for continuing the Sirtfood diet, reviewing your goals allows you to track your diet's progress. Remember that while drawing up your plans, the processes and pathways are also defined. These defined pathways are used to monitor your progress with the Sirtfood diet.

Understand That It Is Acceptable to Make Mistakes

One of the banes of most dieters is cheating or eating off-plan. It occurs when they eat foods that are not in tandem with the dictates of their diet. In the Sirtfood diet, it is possible to eat off-plan too. There are days you may overeat or eat wrongly due to forgetfulness, and some days you may give in to your cravings. If and when any of these occasions, do not be too hard on yourself and do not lose hope. It would help if you remembered that you are only human, and it is acceptable to make mistakes. Most importantly, you must remember that the most vital and helpful step you can take after eating out of the diet is to pick up yourself and learn from your mistakes.

You need to understand the reason for the relapse. Was it due to cravings or forgetfulness? What exactly went wrong? Getting answers to these questions will help you map out the steps that you must take to avoid such relapse afterward. For instance, if the mistake was due to forgetfulness, you can set up periodic reminders to always keep you in check at all times.

On the other hand, if the mistake was born out of cravings, you may need to talk to your dietician. The dietician will help you find out if the craving's food items can hurt the Sirtfood diet plans. It will help provide options and solutions to overcome this mistake.

In summary, after making a mistake with the diet plan, the next course of action should be how to overcome the error and prevent future occurrences.

Combine Exercises with The Sirtfood Diet

Exercises are very beneficial to human health. Combining it with a healthy diet like the Sirtfood diet increases the health benefits that can be derived. However, exercising regularly during the diet has immense health benefits and helps you stay focused on a diet. You may wonder how that works.

By combining exercise with the Sirtfood diet, there is a considerable likelihood of quickly and easily achieving your set goals. For people going into the Sirtfood diet to achieve healthy weight loss, exercising is a great plus that quickly achieves this goal. Also, exercises help you accomplish this accessible for people going into the diet for the energy-boosting effect.

When your set goals are achieved easily during the Sirtfood diet, the zeal to remain focused and maintain the diet is renewed. The possibility of getting discouraged during the dieting process is reduced as you can see the diet's achievements.

Smart Snacking

While on a diet such as the Sirtfood diet, there is a restriction on what to eat and drink. Hence, in situations where you need to be away from home for an extended period, you need to ensure that you have a reliable source of Sirtfoods to eat when the need arises. Because it is not very comfortable to pack food items with you wherever you go, snacks remain the best and most suitable option.

Snacks and fast food are handy in serving as an alternative to real foods when the need arises. However, not all snacks can be used in place of Sirtfoods. It is the origination of the concept of smart snacks. Smart snacks are healthy and appropriate alternatives that can be used in place of Sirtfoods, especially when you are away from home or cannot access your Sirtfood items. Snacking is another way of maintaining the Sirtfood diet. By having smart snacks on you whenever you are far from home, you have the opportunity to feed your body with needed nutrients through the smart snack without eating unhealthy food or out of the Sirtfood diet.

Make the Best Out of Your Restaurant Time

Sometimes, it is impossible to have access to smart snacks. It may be due to forgetfulness on your part, or you cannot afford to get some because of time or space. In most cases, the only option you are left with at this point is to eat out or starve until you get home. Of course, starving yourself is not an ideal option as it undermines your strength to carry out your work and other activities effectively.

The viable choice here is to eat at a restaurant. As discouraging as it may sound to your Sirtfood diet plan, you can still attempt to make the best out of it. Make inquiries about the availability of some Sirtfoods in the restaurant. While some particular foods are peculiar to the Sirtfood diet, some general food items are also sirtuin-friendly. Try to get these foods if you can.

However, if these foods are not available, opt-in for nutritious or healthy foods; although these foods are not Sirtfoods, they are filled with essential nutrients that will do your body a whole lot of good. If these foods and fruits are available at your eat-out spot or restaurant, they are safe for you to eat.

If the restaurants do not have these types of food in stock, you can eat whatever pleases you on the menu. It is the other best option other than starving yourself. However, you remember that you need to balance this episode of eating out with sufficient Sirtfoods so that your goals are not affected.

Mind What You Eat

There is a practice called mindful eating. It involves people paying detailed and intricate attention to what they eat and its effect on their bodies. To some school of thought, mindful eating is a diet with some health benefits. While I will not precisely classify mindful eating as a diet type, there is no doubt that it has some advantages, health-wise. These benefits, among other things, will help you stay focused on your Sirtfood diet.

By practicing mindful eating, the body is put to receive more nutrients and less unhealthy elements. It is because mindful eating requires researching thoroughly into the nutritional constituents of what we eat. By doing so, nutritious and beneficial foods are distinguished from unhealthy food. Since it is unlikely that anyone would knowingly consume unhealthy foods, more nutrients are fed into the body by eating healthy foods.

Feeding the body with enough nutrients helps maintain the Sirtfood diet. With abundant nutrient in the body, the benefits of the diet can easily be achieved and sustained. Therefore, if you wish to maintain the Sirtfood diet, you can practice mindful eating to help with the process.

Stick to The Sirtfood Diet Plan

This point sounds like a no-brainer, but it is crucial and requires reiteration. Sticking to the diet plan is one sure way of ensuring that both short-term and long-term goals of the diet are achieved. Sticking to the diet plan from the inception of the Sirtfood diet is instrumental in attaining the short-term goals. These goals include drastic but healthy weight loss and improvement in the body's energy level, among other things. Apart from their inherent health benefits, the attainment of these goals is a significant boost to anyone's morale under this diet. Seeing that some of the goals set at the beginning of the diet have been achieved, remaining focused and maintaining the diet would be less stressful. Hence sticking to the diet plan is a vital step in ensuring that you retain the Sirtfood diet.

Furthermore, the success of all the tips recently given is dependent on your ability to stick with the diet plan. Without the determination to stick to the diet plan, all the other suggestions will be useless and ineffective.

These tips given help you maintain the zeal and momentum for the Sirtfood diet. This way, the successful completion of the dieting process is ensured.

chapter 1 ... Breakfast...

Kale & Orange Juice

Preparation time: 10 minutes

Cooking time: 0 minutes

Servings: 2

Ingredients:

- 5 large oranges, peeled and sectioned
- 2 bunches fresh kale

Directions:

1. Add all ingredients into a juicer and extract. Pour into 2 glasses and serve immediately.

Nutrition:

Calories: 197

Carbs: 49g

Fat: 2g

Protein: 0g

1. Tropical Chocolate Delight

Preparation time: 30 minutes

Cooking time: 0 minutes

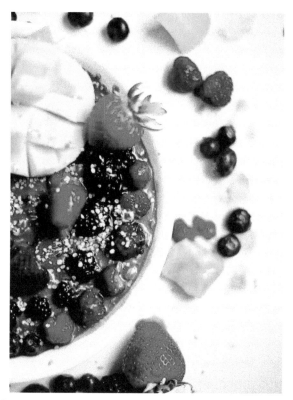

Servings: 1

Ingredients

- 1 mango, peeled & de-stoned
- 3oz fresh pineapple, chopped

- 2oz kale

- 1oz arugula

- 1 tablespoon 100% cocoa powder or cacao nibs

- 5fl oz coconut milk

Directions:

1. Put all of the fixings into a blender and blitz until smooth. You can add a little water if it seems too thick.

Nutrition:

Calories: 90

Carbs: 3g

Fat: 2g

Protein: 16g

2. Walnut & Spiced Apple Tonic

Preparation time: 30 minutes

Cooking time: 0 minutes

Servings: 1

Ingredients:

- 6 walnuts halves

- 1 apple, cored

- 1 banana

- ½ teaspoon matcha powder

- ½ teaspoon cinnamon

- Pinch of ground nutmeg

Directions:

1. Put all of the fixings into a blender and add sufficient water to cover them. Blitz until smooth and creamy.

Nutrition:

Calories: 126

Carbs: 15g

Fat: 7g Protein: 2g

3. Classic French Toast

Preparation time: 10 minutes

Cooking time: 45 minutes

Servings: 2

Ingredients:

- 4 huge eggs

- 1/2 cup entire milk

- 1 teaspoon vanilla concentrate

- 1/2 teaspoons ground cinnamon partitioned

- 8 cuts Brioche bread

Directions:

1. On the off chance that is utilizing an electric iron, preheat the frying pan to 350 degrees F. Race until very much consolidated.

2. Plunge each side of the bread in the egg blend. Soften a little margarine on the hot frying pan or in a large skillet over medium warmth. Serve the French toast warm with maple syrup, powdered sugar, and berries, whenever wanted.

Nutrition:

Calories: 251

Carbs: 37g

Fat: 5g

Protein: 13g

4. Simple Tofu Scramble

Preparation time: 10 minutes

Cooking Time: 30 minutes

Servings 4

Ingredients:

Tofu scramble:

- 16 ounces of extra firm tofu
- 4 cups kale, loosely chopped
- ½ red onion, thinly sliced
- 1 red pepper, thinly sliced
- Extra virgin olive oil

Sauce:

- 1 tsp garlic powder
- 1 tsp cumin powder
- 1/2 tsp chili powder
- 1 tsp sea salt
- 1/2 tsp turmeric (optional)

Directions:

1. Make sure that the tofu is drained. You can do this using an absorbent towel with a skillet on top. Do this for about 10-15 minutes.

2. In a small bowl, prepare the sauce by adding all the dry spices and then add enough water to become a pourable sauce. Set aside.

3. Over medium heat, use a large skillet, and add about 2 tbsp. Of extra virgin olive oil once the skillet is hot. Add the red pepper and onion, then season with salt and pepper. Stir and cook for about 3-5 minutes.

4. Add the kale and season to taste with salt and pepper. Cover it for another 2 minutes. Unwrap the tofu, then crumble into bite-sizes using a fork or a spoon.

5. Move the veggies on one side of the pan, then add the tofu to the clear spot. Sauté for about 2-3 minutes, then pour in the sauce over the tofu.

6. Stir and cook until the tofu is lightly browned. Serve and enjoy. You can also add more sirtuin-rich food on the side.

Nutrition:

Calories: 220

Carbs: 15g

Fat: 8g

Protein: 25g

5. Strawberry, Rocket (Arugula) & Feta Salad

Preparation time: 5 Minutes

Cooking Time: 50 Minutes

Servings: 4

Ingredients

- 75g arugula leaves

- 3oz feta cheese, crumbled

- 3½ oz strawberries halved

- 8 walnut halves

- 2 tablespoons flaxseeds

Directions:

1. Mix all the fixing in a bowl, then scatter them onto two plates. For an extra sirt food boost, you can drizzle over some olive oil.

Nutrition:

Calories: 118

Carbs: 7g

Fat: 9g / Protein: 4 g

6. Mushroom Courgetti & Lemon Caper Pesto

Preparation time: 5 Minutes

Cooking Time: 25 Minutes

Servings: 4

Ingredients

- 4 courgettes (zucchinis)
- 10 oyster mushrooms, sliced
- 1 red onion, sliced
- 2 tablespoons olive oil
- 2 tablespoons lemon caper pesto
- 50g arugula leaves

Directions

1. Spiralize the courgettes into spaghetti. If you don't have a spiralizer, finely cut the vegetables lengthways into long 'spaghetti' strips.

2. Heat-up olive oil in a frying pan, add the mushrooms and onions, and cook for minutes. Add in the courgettes and the pesto and cook for 5 minutes. Scatter the arugula leaves onto plates and serve the courgettes on top. Serve.

Nutrition:

Calories: 245

Carbs: 0g : Fat 17g

7. Mushroom Scrambled Eggs

Preparation time: 10 minutes

Cooking time: 20 minutes

Servings: 1

Ingredients

- 1 teaspoon ground garlic

- 1 teaspoon mild curry powder

- 20g lettuce, approximately sliced

- 1 teaspoon extra virgin olive oil

- 1/2 bird's eye peeled, thinly chopped

- A couple of mushrooms, finely chopped

- 5g parsley, finely chopped

- Optional - insert a seed mix for a topper plus some rooster sauce for taste

Directions:

1. Mix the curry and garlic powder, and then add just a little water until you've achieved a light glue. Steam the lettuce for 2 - 3 minutes.

2. Heat the oil in a skillet over moderate heat and fry the chili and mushrooms 2-3 minutes until they've begun to soften and brown.

3. Insert the eggs and spice paste, cook over moderate heat, add the carrot, and then cook over medium heat for a further minute. In the end, put in the parsley, mix well and serve.

Nutrition:

Calories: 102

Carbs: 5g

Fat: 5g

Protein: 11g

8. Blue Hawaii Smoothie

Preparation time: 10 minutes

Cooking time: 20 minutes

Servings: 1

Ingredients:

- 2 tablespoons ring s or approximately 4-5 balls
- 1/2 cup frozen tomatoes
- 2 tbsp ground flaxseed
- 1/8 cup tender coconut (unsweetened, organic)
- Few walnuts
- 1/2 cup fat-free yogurt
- 5-6 ice cubes
- Splash of water

Directions:

1. Throw all of the ingredients together and combine until smooth. You might need to shake it or put more water in the mix. Serve,

Nutrition:

Calories: 221

Carbs: 43g

Fat: 3g

Protein: 5g

9. Moroccan Spiced Eggs

Preparation time: 1 hour

Cooking time: 50 minutes

Servings: 2

Ingredients:

- 1 tsp olive oil
- 1 shallot, stripped and finely hacked
- 1 red (chime) pepper, deseeded and finely hacked
- 1 garlic clove, stripped and finely hacked
- 1 courgette (zucchini), stripped and finely hacked
- 1 tbsp tomato puree (glue)
- ½ tsp gentle stew powder
- ¼ tsp ground cinnamon
- ¼ tsp ground cumin
- ½ tsp salt
- 1 × 400g (14oz) can hacked tomatoes
- 1 x 400g (14oz) may chickpeas in water
- a little bunch of level leaf parsley (10g (1/3oz)), cleaved

- 4 medium eggs at room temperature

Directions:

1. Heat the oil in a pan, include the shallot and red (ringer) pepper, and fry delicately for 5 minutes. At that point, put the garlic and courgette (zucchini) and cook for one more moment or two. Include the tomato puree (glue), flavors, and salt and mix through.

2. Add the cleaved tomatoes and chickpeas and increment the warmth to medium. On top of the dish, stew the sauce for 30 minutes.

3. Remove from the warmth and mix in the cleaved parsley. Preheat the grill to 350F. When you are prepared to cook the eggs, bring the tomato sauce up to a delicate stew and move to a little broiler confirmation dish.

4. Crack the eggs on the dish and lower them delicately into the stew. Spread with thwart and prepare in the grill for 10-15 minutes. Serve the blend in unique dishes with the eggs coasting on the top.

Nutrition:

Calories: 417

Carbs: 38g

Fat: 24g / Protein: 18g

10. Chilaquiles with Gochujang

Preparation time: 30 minutes

Cooking time: 20 minutes

Servings: 2

Ingredients:

- 1 dried ancho chili
- 2 cups of water
- 1 cup squashed tomatoes
- 2 cloves of garlic
- 1 teaspoon genuine salt
- 1/2 tablespoons gochujang
- 5 to 6 cups tortilla chips
- 3 enormous eggs
- 1 tablespoon olive oil

Directions:

1. Get the water to heat a pot. Add the anchor Chile to the bubbled water and drench for 15 minutes to give it an opportunity to stout up.

2. When completed, use tongs or a spoon to extricate Chile. Make sure to spare the water for the sauce.

3. Mix the doused Chile, 1 cup of saved high temp water, squashed tomatoes, garlic, salt, and gochujang until smooth.

4. Empty sauce into a large dish and warmth over medium warmth for 4 to 5 minutes. Mood killer the heat and include the tortilla chips. Mix the chips to cover with the sauce.

5. In a different skillet, shower a teaspoon of oil and fry an egg on top until the whites have settled. Plate the egg and cook the remainder of the eggs.

6. Top the chips with the seared eggs, cotija, hacked cilantro, jalapeños, onions, and avocado. Serve right away.

Nutrition:

Calories: 443

Carbs: 32g

Fat: 32g

Protein: 10g

11. Twice Baked Breakfast Potatoes

Preparation time: 1 hour 10 minutes

Cooking time: 1 hour

Servings: 2

Ingredients:

- 2 medium reddish-brown potatoes, cleaned and pricked with a fork everywhere
- 2 tablespoons unsalted spread
- 3 tablespoons overwhelming cream
- 4 rashers cooked bacon
- 4 huge eggs
- ½ cup destroyed cheddar
- Daintily cut chives
- Salt and pepper to taste

Directions:

1. Preheat grill to 400 F. Spot potatoes straightforwardly on stove rack in the grill's focal point and prepare for 30 to 45 minutes.

40

2.   Evacuate and permit potatoes to cool for around 15 minutes. Cut every potato down the middle longwise and burrow every half out, scooping the potato substance into a blending bowl.

3.   Gather margarine and cream to the potato and pound into a single unit until smooth — season with salt and pepper and mix.

4.   Spread a portion of the potato blend into each emptied potato skin base and sprinkle with one tablespoon cheddar.

5.   Add one rasher bacon to every half and top with a raw egg. Spot potatoes onto a heating sheet and come back to the appliance.

6.   Lower broiler temperature to 375F and heat potatoes until egg whites simply set and yolks are as yet runny.

7.   Top every potato with a sprinkle of the rest of the cheddar, season with salt and pepper, and finish with cut chives.

Nutrition:

Calories: 175

Carbs: 32g

Fat: 1g .Protein: 10g

12. Sirt Muesli

Preparation time: 15 minutes

Cooking time: 0 minutes

Servings: 1

Ingredients:

- A 1-quarter cup of buckwheat flakes

- 2/3 cup of buckwheat puffs

- 3 tbsp. coconut flakes

- 1-quarter cup Medjool dates

- 1/8 cup of chopped walnuts

- 1 1/2 tbsp. of cocoa nibs

- 2/3 cup of chopped strawberries

- 3/8 cup plain Greek Yoghurt

Directions:

1. Simply mix all the ingredients in a clean bowl, and enjoy the great goodness of this delicacy. However, only add strawberries and yogurt when you are ready to eat.

Nutrition:

Calories: 368

Carbs: 54g

Fat: 16g

Protein: 26g

13. Sirtfood Omelet

Preparation time: 15 minutes

Cooking time: 10 minutes

Servings: 2

Ingredients:

- 3 medium-sized eggs
- 1 and a 1-quarter oz. sliced red endive
- 2 tbsp. chopped parsley
- 1 tsp. turmeric
- 1 tsp. extra virgin olive oil

Directions:

1. Wipe your pan clean and then pour in some oil – enough to cook the three eggs. Beat your eggs thoroughly and add in the turmeric, parsley, and endive.

2. Pour in oil into your pan and heat at medium heat. Pour the egg mixture in the hot oil and move the mixture around with a spatula.

3. Swirl the mixture around the pan. Adjust the heat to low, then allow the omelet to firm up and even out at the edges. Fold your omelet in half, roll it up and serve hot.

Nutrition:

Calories: 210

Carbs: 1g

Fat: 5g

Protein: 6g

14. Yogurt, Berries, Walnuts, And Dark Chocolate

Preparation time: 15 minutes

Cooking time: 0 minutes

Servings: 2

Ingredients:

- 25 grams of mixed berries

- 2/3 cup of plain Greek yogurt

- ¼ cup of walnuts

- 10g of dark chocolate (85% pure cocoa)

Directions:

1. Get a clean bowl and add in your berries. Pour the plain Greek yogurt over the berries. Add in your walnuts and dark chocolate, and food is ready.

Nutrition:

Calories: 180

Carbs: 12g

Fat: 14g

Protein: 3g

15. Miso and Sesame Glazed Tofu with Ginger and Chili Stir

Preparation time: 15 minutes

Cooking time: 35 minutes

Servings: 3

Ingredients:

- 1 tbsp mirin
- 20 grams of miso paste
- 150 grams of tofu
- 40 grams of celery
- 40 grams of red onion
- 120 grams of zucchini
- 1 piece of Thai chili
- 2 cloves of garlic
- 1 teaspoon of fresh ginger (finely chopped)
- 50 grams of kale
- 2 teaspoons of sesame seeds
- 35 grams of buckwheat
- 1 teaspoon of ground turmeric

- 2 teaspoons of extra virgin olive oil

- 1 teaspoon of tamari sauce

Directions:

1. Heat your oven to four hundred degrees. Get a small roasting pan and line it with parchment paper. Combine the mirin and the miso. Slice up your tofu lengthwise, and then make each piece out into a triangular shape.

2. Spread the miso mixture over the tofu and allow the tofu to get steeped in the mix. Cut up your celery, red onion, and zucchini, then cut up the chili, garlic, and ginger.

3. Allow the kale to cook in a steamer for 5 minutes gently, then transfer your tofu into the roasting pan and spread the sesame seeds over it. Allow the mixture to roast in the oven for 20 minutes.

4. Rinse your buckwheat, and then sieve. Bring a pan filled with water to boil and add in the turmeric. Cook the buckwheat noodles and strain.

5. Allow the oil to heat in a frying pan, and then add the celery, onion, zucchini, chili, garlic, and ginger. Allow the entire mix to fry on high heat for 2 minutes. Reduce the heat to medium for 4 minutes until the vegetables are cooked.

6. Add a tablespoon of water if the vegetables get stuck to the pan. Spread in the kale and tamari and allow the

mixture to cook for another minute. Serve the cooked tofu with the greens and the buckwheat.

Nutrition:

Calories: 165

Carbs: 15g

Fat: 8g

Protein: 10g

16. Buckwheat Pancakes, Mushrooms, Red Onions, And Kale Salad

Preparation time: 15 minutes

Cooking time: 10 minutes

Servings: 4

Ingredients:

- 1 buckwheat pancake

- 50g button mushrooms

- 15 grams of chicken

- 200g Kale

- 20g red onions

- Extra Virgin Olive Oil

Directions:

1. Clean and cut the button mushrooms. Clean and cut the kale into thin strips and the red onions into rings. Combine the green cabbage and onion in a bowl, season with a drizzle of olive oil and possibly a little lemon.

2. Cut the chicken into pieces. In a pan, arrange a drizzle of olive oil and add the chicken pieces. Add the

mushrooms and brown them. Place everything in the buckwheat pancake, and close the pancake.

3. On a plate, arrange the green cabbage or red onion salad, then place the hot buckwheat pancake beside it. Enjoy your meal!

Nutrition:

Calories: 320

Carbs: 29g

Fat: 2g

Protein: 7g

17. Naan Bread with Baked Tofu and Cauliflower

Preparation time: 15 minutes

Cooking time: 60 minutes

Servings: 2

Ingredients:

- 50 g firm plain tofu
- 50 g cauliflower
- ½ clove garlic
- ½ small onion
- 50ml of water
- 50ml coconut milk
- ½ tablespoon of tomato puree
- ½ teaspoon powdered Indian broth
- ½ tablespoon coconut oil
- ½ teaspoon curry powder
- ½ teaspoon cumin
- ½ tablespoon potato starch

Naan bread:

- 75g wheat flour

- 1 plain yogurt

- 2 pinches of sugar

- 5g baker's yeast or 8 g dehydrated yeast

- 5g salt

- 2 tablespoons extra virgin olive oil

- 5 cl lukewarm water

- 1 teaspoon caraway seed

Directions:

1. Peel and mince the garlic and the onions. In a casserole dish, sauté everything in coconut oil with the curry and cumin until lightly colored.

2. Add the coconut milk, the tomato puree, 50 ml of water, and the Indian broth. Mix well, then bring to a delicate simmer. Add the tofu pieces and the cauliflower.

3. Cook gently without the lid on for about 20 minutes until the cauliflower is slightly tender. Dilute the starch with a little cooking juice, then pour back into the casserole dish and continue cooking for 5 minutes. Serve with basmati rice and naan bread.

4. For the naan bread, put the flour in your food processor. Add the crumbled yeast, olive oil, sugar, yogurt, caraway seeds, and mix well.

5. Proceed by adding the water and continue mixing with the whisk until the dough is soft and comes off your bowl's sides.

6. Now place the ball of dough in a small bowl, then cover, and allow to stand for 30 minutes. Heat an empty pan, and cook the naan bread on each side for four minutes to remove moisture. Enjoy your mouth-watering delicacy.

Nutrition:

Calories: 130

Carbs: 22g

Fat: 4g

Protein: 4g

18. Date and Walnut Strawberry Porridge

Preparation time: 15 minutes

Cooking time: 10 minutes

Servings: 2

Ingredients:

- 2 Medjool dates – chopped

- 200 ml of milk

- 35 grams buckwheat flakes

- Walnut – 4 chopped halves

- 50 grams strawberries – hulled

Directions:

1. Pour the milk into a cooking pot and add the chopped dates. Stir in well and allow the milk to heat up on medium heat. Add the buckwheat flakes, then stir to combine.

2. Cook the flakes with occasional stirring to your preferred consistency. Add walnuts and stir in to combine. Top with cherries when served and enjoy your sirtfood breakfast.

Nutrition:

Calories: 137

Fat: 2.5 g

Carbs: 27 g

Protein: 3 g

19. Chia and Almonds Blueberry Bowl

Preparation time: 15 minutes

Cooking time: 0 minutes

Servings: 3

Ingredients:

- 1/8 cup blueberries

- 2 Medjool dates

- 3/8 cup coconut milk

- ½ tablespoon almond butter

- 1/8 cup buckwheat groats - raw

- 1/4 teaspoon cardamom - powdered

- ½ tablespoon cocoa nibs

- Pinch of salt

- ½ tablespoon almonds

- 1/8 cup chia seeds

Directions:

1. Combine coconut milk with dates, cardamom, salt, and almond butter and place the combined ingredients into a blender. Blend until the mixture is smooth.

2. Combine chia seeds and buckwheat groats in a bowl, then add the blended mixture to the bowl and stir to combine.

3. Cover the bowl and let it rest in the fridge for at least 15 minutes. Top the bowl delight with almonds, cocoa nibs, and blueberries.

Nutrition:

Calories: 243

Fat: 16 g

Carbs: 25 g

Protein: 12 g

20. Chocolate Buckwheat Porridge

Preparation time: 15 minutes

Cooking time: 15 minutes

Servings: 2

Ingredients:

- ½ cup of buckwheat groats – raw, soaked overnight, rinsed and drained of water
- ¾ cup of milk – plant-based would work better in the spirit of the diet
- ¼ cup of milk – for topping
- 1 tablespoon of cocoa - powdered
- 5 strawberries – mashed
- 1 tablespoon pecan nuts
- ¼ cup blueberries
- 1 tablespoon coconut flakes

Directions:

1. Add the ¾ of milk to the saucepan together with mashed strawberries, cocoa powder, and buckwheat groats.

2. Cook on low, medium heat for 12 to 15 minutes while frequently stirring until the buckwheat is cooked according to your personal preferences.

3. Add more milk, if necessary, during cooking from the cup of milk reserved for topping. Top with pecan nuts, more milk, blueberries, and coconut flakes.

Nutrition:

Calories: 167

Fat: 1 g

Carbs: 33 g

Protein: 5.5 g

21. Mushroom and Buckwheat Breakfast Bowl

Preparation time: 15 minutes

Cooking time: 15 minutes

Servings: 4

Ingredients:

- 2 tablespoons butter
- 2 cups buckwheat groats – toasted
- 8 chestnut mushrooms
- 1 onion – medium, chopped
- 3 sprigs of parsley – flat-leaf
- Pinch of salt
- 1 teaspoon oregano
- 1 boiled egg per serving

Directions:

1. Put the buckwheat in a cooking pot and add the water and salt. Cook until the water evaporates, and the buckwheat is soft. Remove from the stove and cover the pot.

2. Let the buckwheat rest for an additional 15 minutes. In the meanwhile, heat a pan and add the butter. Once the butter is melted, add sliced mushrooms and chopped onions and caramelize while occasionally stirring.

3. Add the chopped parsley once the mushrooms are browned and sauté for 5 minutes. Add the buckwheat and stir in to combine with the rest of the ingredients.

4. Lastly, add oregano while cooking for two more minutes. Top with a boiled egg and serve while warm.

Nutrition:

Calories: 204

Fat: 3 g

Carbs: 34 g

Protein: 8 g

22. Spring Quinoa Salad

Preparation time: 15 minutes

Cooking time: 20 minutes

Servings: 2

Ingredients:

- 1 cucumber – peeled, sliced
- 1 tomato – chopped in large chunks
- 1 avocado – peeled and chopped
- 1 cup quinoa uncooked
- 2 cups of water
- ¼ large red onion – chopped
- 5 grams parsley – chopped
- 1 tablespoon extra-virgin olive oil
- 1 large egg – cooked
- Salt to taste

Directions:

1. Take a small saucepan and pour two cups of water along with one cup of quinoa. Bring quinoa and water to a boil, then cover the saucepan and set the heat to low medium.

2. Cook for 20 minutes or until the water is reduced. Let quinoa cool for a while as you chop and slice the veggies and parsley.

3. Add the veggies and parsley to quinoa, then add a tablespoon of olive oil. Stir well to combine, then top with sliced cooked egg.

Nutrition:

Calories: 407

Fat: 7 g

Carbs: 35 g

Protein: 9 g

23. Apple and Blackcurrant Pancakes

Preparation time: 15 minutes

Cooking time: 20 minutes

Servings: 4

Ingredients:

- 125 grams flour – plain
- 1 teaspoon baking powder
- 2 tablespoons caster sugar
- ½ teaspoon salt
- 2 apples – peeled and cut into small pieces
- 300 ml milk – semi-skimmed
- 75 grams porridge oats
- 2 egg whites
- 2 teaspoons light olive oil

Sauce:

- 120 grams blackcurrants
- 2 tablespoons caster sugar
- 3 tablespoons water

Directions:

1. Prepare the ingredients for the pancake sauce. Place the blackcurrants and sugar in a small pan. Pour water into the pan and cook the sauce for 10 or 15 minutes after bringing it to a simmer.

2. As the sauce is cooking, take a large bowl and place all the dry ingredients sugar, oats, baking powder, and salt. Mix to combine, then add apples and start adding milk, a little at a time, as you are whisking the mixture.

3. Mix the egg whites in a separate bowl, then add the whisked whites to the pancake mixture. Heat a pancake pan and add ½ tablespoon of the oil.

4. Pour a quarter of batter, one at the time, baking pancakes until golden brown on both sides. Repeat the process until you make four pancakes. Serve with the sauce on top.

Nutrition:

Calories: 337

Fat: 7 g

Carbs: 20 g

Protein: 4 g

24. Breakfast Shakshuka

Preparation time: 15 minutes

Cooking time: 20 minutes

Servings: 3

Ingredients:

- 1 tablespoon extra-virgin olive oil
- 40 grams red onion – chopped
- 1 garlic clove – chopped
- 30 grams celery – chopped
- 1 bird's eye chili – sliced
- 400 grams tomatoes – tinned, chopped
- 1 tablespoon chopped parsley
- 30 grams kale – chopped
- 1 teaspoon cumin – ground
- 1 teaspoon turmeric – ground
- 1 teaspoon paprika - ground
- 2 eggs

Directions:

1. Heat a small deep pan on low-medium heat. Add the olive oil, then add garlic, onions, chili, celery, and spices. Cook for 2 minutes or until mildly softened.

2. Add tomatoes to the mixture and stir well to combine the ingredients. Simmer the sauce on low heat while occasionally stirring not to let the sauce burn. Add kale and cook for 5 more minutes.

3. In case the sauce appears to be too thick, add some water to reduce it. Once the sauce reaches the right consistency, add parsley and stir in well.

4. Reduce the heat to low, then make two holes in the sauce. Crack the eggs, one in each sauce hole, then cover the pan with the lid and cook for 10 to 12 minutes. Serve hot, and eat right from the pan ideally.

Nutrition:

Calories: 309

Fat: 34 g

Carbs: 22 g

Protein: 23 g

25. Buckwheat Pancakes with Dark Chocolate Sauce

Preparation time: 15 minutes

Cooking time: 15 minutes

Servings: 6

Ingredients:

- 350 ml of milk

- 150 grams buckwheat flour

- 1 tablespoon extra-virgin olive oil

- 1 egg

Sauce:

- 1 tablespoon double cream

- 85 ml of milk

- 100 grams dark chocolate – 85% cocoa

Toppings:

- 400 grams of strawberries

- 100 grams walnuts

Directions:

1. Place all the ingredients for making pancakes into a blender except the oil. Blend buckwheat flour, milk, and the egg until the batter is smooth.

2. Leave the mixture aside and start making the chocolate sauce. Bring a pot of water to a boil, then place a heatproof bowl on the top of the pot.

3. Add chocolate to the bowl and use a spatula to stir as you are melting the chocolate.

4. Add double cream and olive oil to the melted chocolate and mix well to combine. Heat a frying pan until it starts to smoke, then add the oil.

5. In case the pan is hot enough, it will only take 1 minute for each side to get the pancake done. Put some of the batters into the pan and fry on both sides.

6. Once both sides are done, add some strawberries on the top and roll up the pancake. Serve with the dark chocolate sauce.

Nutrition:

Calories: 143

Fat: 8 g

Carbs: 15 g

Protein: 4 g

26. Banana and Blueberry Oat Pancakes

Preparation time: 15 minutes

Cooking time: 5 minutes

Servings: 6

Ingredients:

- 6 bananas

- 6 eggs

- 150 grams oats – rolled

- 2 teaspoons baking powder

- ¼ teaspoon salt

- 25 grams blueberries

- 1-2 tablespoons of coconut oil

Directions:

1. Pulse the rolled oats around 1 minute or until oats are turned into flour. Add bananas, baking powder, salt, eggs, and pulse for 2 minutes or until the batter turns smooth.

2. Add blueberries and leave the mixture to rest for around 10 minutes for the baking powder to activate. Heat-up a frying pan and add some oil.

3. Once the oil is heated, add some pancake mix to form a pancake. Fry on medium-high heat. Fry on both sides until golden brown. Enjoy your breakfast.

Nutrition:

Calories: 187

Fat: 3 g

Carbs: 33 g

Protein: 6 g

27. Turmeric Pancakes with Lemon Yoghurt

Preparation time: 15 minutes

Cooking time: 6 minutes

Servings: 8

Ingredients:

- 2 teaspoons turmeric - ground
- 1 ½ teaspoon cumin – ground
- 1 teaspoon salt
- 1 teaspoon coriander – ground
- ½ teaspoon garlic powder
- ½ teaspoon freshly ground black pepper
- 1 head broccoli – florets, cut
- 2 tablespoons unsweetened plain almond milk
- 1 cup almond flour
- 3 eggs
- 2 tablespoons coconut oil

Sauce:

- 1 cup yogurt – Greek, plain

- 1 garlic clove – minced

- 2 tablespoons lemon juice

- ½ teaspoons turmeric – ground

- 10 mint leaves – fresh

- 2 teaspoons lemon zest

Directions:

1. First, you will make yogurt sauce as you want it to cool properly before serving. Mix all the fixing from the list for the sauce in a bowl. Mix to combine and place the sauce in the fridge.

2. Get ready to make the pancake batter. Add coriander, garlic, turmeric, salt, cumin, and pepper to a separate bowl. Cut the broccoli head and place the florets into the food processor. Pulse until you get grainy texture-out of the broccoli. Place broccoli florets in the bowl with spices and herbs and mix well. Add almond milk and flour to the mixture.

3. Lightly beat the 3 eggs, then transfer the eggs to the bowl with the ingredients. Stir to combine all the ingredients.

4. Heat a frying pan on medium-low heat and add coconut oil. Once the oil is heated, pour a quarter of the batter into the pan. Fry from 2 to 3 minutes on each side until pancakes turns golden brown.

5. Repeat the process three more times until the batter is gone. Serve with cold yogurt sauce and enjoy!

Nutrition:

Calories: 124

Fat: 3.5 g

Carbs: 10 g / protein 1.7g

28. Buckwheat Pancakes with Pineapple

Preparation time: 15 minutes

Cooking time: 6 minutes

Servings: 4

Ingredients:

- 1/ 4 cup almond flour
- 1 cup buckwheat flour
- 2 tablespoons hemp seeds
- 1 teaspoon baking powder
- ¼ teaspoon salt
- ½ teaspoon allspice
- 150 grams of cottage cheese
- 1 teaspoon vanilla extract
- 2 tablespoons maple syrup
- 1 egg
- 1 cup almond milk – unsweetened
- 1 small pineapple - cut into rings, peeled and cored
- 2 tablespoons coconut oil

Directions:

1. Combine all dry ingredients from the list and mix well in a mixing bowl. Make sure not to leave out the hemp seeds.

2. Add vanilla, cottage cheese, maple syrup, and an egg. Start adding milk little by little as you are whisking the mixture. Whisk until you get a homogenous mass.

3. Set the stove to medium heat and heat the pancake pan or griddle. Add one to two tablespoons of coconut oil and once the oil is heated, add a slice of pineapple.

4. Pour some of the pancake batters over the pineapple ring—Bake for 3 minutes on each side. Repeat the process with the remaining batter. Serve and enjoy!

Nutrition:

Calories: 316

Fat: 13 g

Carbs: 42 g

Protein: 12 g

29. Egg Whites and Pepper Omelet

Preparation time: 15 minutes

Cooking time: 10 minutes

Servings: 1

Ingredients:

- 4 egg whites
- 1 cup red bell pepper - diced
- 1 cup yellow bell pepper - diced
- 1/8 cup red onion – diced
- Salt to taste
- ½ bird's eye chili - sliced
- ½ tablespoon extra-virgin olive oil

Directions:

1. Heat-up a skillet and add the oil. Whisk the egg whites and discard the yolks, whisk until smooth, then add some salt.

2. Combine with peppers and onions, then whisk until thoroughly combined. Pour the mixture into the skillet and cook on medium heat.

3. Ensure that the eggs are settled and cooked before folding the omelet with a spatula to make a roll. Serve.

Nutrition:

Calories: 223

Fat: 10 g

Carbs: 16 g- Protein 18g

30. Baked Apples

Preparation time: 15 minutes

Cooking time: 40 minutes

Servings: 1

Ingredients:

- 1 large apple
- 1 tablespoon brown sugar blend
- ¼ teaspoon cinnamon
- 1 Medjool date - chopped
- ½ tablespoon chopped walnuts
- 1/ 4 tablespoon olive oil butter
- ½ cup of water

Directions:

1. Warm oven to 350 degrees F. Remove the core to the bottom but leave the bottom. Prepare a small baking dish and

line it with parchment.

2. Remove the seeds and use a spoon to get rid of the excess insides. Take a small bowl and combine sugar with cinnamon, walnuts, and dates. Top with butter.

3. Place a cup of water in the baking dish with the apple. Bake for 30 to 40 minutes until the apple tenders. Leave it to rest for 10 minutes and enjoy!

Nutrition:

Calories: 242

Fat: 8 g

Carbs: 44 g

Protein: 1 g

31. Plum Yoghurt Bowl with Coconut and Cocoa Nibs

Preparation time: 15 minutes

Cooking time: 0 minutes

Servings: 1

Ingredients:

- 200 g yogurt, natural 1.8%

- 100 g blue plums

- 10 g cocoa nibs

- 10 g peanuts

- 20 g toasted coconut chips

- Agave syrup as needed

Directions:

1. Wash the plums, put a few aside for the topping, divide the rest in two, and remove the stones. Put the pitted plums with the yogurt in a tall mixing vessel and puree finely with the hand blender.

2. Depending on the plums' sweetness, sweeten the mixture with agave syrup, then place it in a bowl. Roughly chop the peanuts and garnish with the remaining plums, cocoa nibs, and coconut chips on the plum yogurt bowl.

Nutrition:

Calories 435

Protein 27 g

Fat 10 g

Carbohydrates 16 g

32. Muesli with Yogurt and Fruits

Preparation time: 15 minutes

Cooking time: 30 minutes

Servings: 2

Ingredients:

- 200 g Greek yogurt

- 50 g strawberries

- 1 medium kiwi

- 25 g almonds

- 25 g peanuts

- 10 g fresh walnuts

- 10 g sunflower seeds

- 10 g coconut flour

- 1 egg white

- 1 tsp xylitol

- ½ teaspoon of ground bourbon vanilla

- 1 pinch of sea salt

Directions:

1. Crush the nuts in the grinder, but do not grind them. Alternatively, chop roughly the nuts with a suitable knife. Put the sunflower seeds, nuts, flour, xylitol, vanilla, salt, and egg white in a bowl and mix well.

2. Sprinkle the muesli mixture on a baking sheet lined with baking paper and spread out. Roast the muesli on the middle rack in the preheated oven at 125 ° C for 20 - 30 minutes.

3. In between, take out the tray two or three times and stir the muesli with a spoon to cooks evenly until golden. Then let the muesli cool down and divide into two glasses or keep airtight until eaten.

4. Peel the kiwi and cut into pieces. Wash the strawberries, let them drain and cut out the stalk, then cut in two. Place the yogurt on the muesli and decorate with the fruits.

Nutrition:

Calories 390

Protein 14 g

Fat 9 g

Carbohydrates 10 g

33. Lime Cream with Peach

Preparation time: 15 minutes

Cooking time: 0 minutes

Servings: 2

Ingredients:

- 200 g quark (lean)

- 300 g yogurt, natural 1.8%

- 1 fresh lime

- 120 g fresh yellow peach

- 1 teaspoon agave syrup

Directions:

1. Rinse and dry the lime with hot water. Use the grater to cut off the lime zest. Then cut the lime in two and squeeze out one half.

2. Wash and drain the peaches. Then split the peaches in two, remove the core and cut into pieces.

3. Put the yogurt and quark in a bowl and mix. Add lime juice and zest and stir in. If required, sweeten the lime cream with agave syrup and pour it into two glasses. Drape the peach pieces on the lime cream and serve.

Nutrition:

Calories 201

Protein 20 g

Fat 3 g

Carbohydrates 16 g

34. Greek Yogurt with Chia and Blueberries

Preparation time: 15 minutes

Cooking time: 0 minutes

Servings: 1

Ingredients:

150 Greek yogurts

- 50 g blueberries

- 2 tbsp chia seeds

- ½ tsp agave syrup (optional)

Directions:

1. Pour Greek yogurt and chia seeds into a bowl and mix. Sweeten the yogurt with a little agave syrup if you like.

2. Wash the blueberries and let them dry in the colander. Put the yogurt in a glass or bowl and drape blueberries on top.

Nutrition:

Calories 297

Protein 9 g

Fat 6 g Carbohydrates 12 g

35. Chia Coconut Pudding with Raspberries

Preparation time: 15 minutes

Cooking time: 0 minutes

Servings: 2

Ingredients:

- 60 g chia seeds
- 500 ml coconut milk (alternatively almond or soy milk)
- 150 g raspberries (fresh or frozen)
- 1 kiwi
- 2 - 3 stalks of fresh mint
- 1 teaspoon agave syrup

Directions:

1. Wash the raspberries and puree about 2/3 of them with the hand blender. Put the chia seeds into the milk, then mix until no more lumps can be seen.

2. Mix the raspberry puree and agave syrup with the chia pudding and whisk well. Let the chia pudding soak in the refrigerator for at least 30 minutes, or better overnight.

3. Peel the kiwi and cut into pieces, then chop the mint and mix with the kiwi. Place the fruit on top of the chia pudding and garnish with mint leaves.

Nutrition:

Calories 396

Protein 11 g

Fat 17 g

Carbohydrates 11 g

36. Plum Yogurt

Preparation time: 15 minutes

Cooking time: 1 minute

Servings: 2

Ingredients:

- ½ lemon
- 1 banana
- 100 g blue plums
- 20 g walnuts (1 heaped tablespoon)
- 1 teaspoon sesame oil
- 2 teaspoons of liquid honey
- 300 g yogurt (1.5% fat)
- ½ teaspoon ground anise

Directions:

1. Squeeze the lemon half. Remove the banana from the peel, cut into slices and moisten with 1 teaspoon of lemon juice. Peel and core the plums and cut the soft flesh into pieces. Chop roughly the walnuts.

2. In a nonstick pan, let the sesame oil heat up slowly. Fry the plums and banana in it for about 1 minute over

medium heat, stirring. Then divide into 2 small bowls and let cool for 5–10 minutes.

3. Whisk the honey, yogurt, and aniseed together. Drizzle over the cooled fruit. Top with the chopped walnuts and serve.

Nutrition:

Calories 258

Protein 8 g

Fat 10 g

Carbohydrates 32 g

37. Berry Bowl

Preparation time: 15 minutes

Cooking time: 10 minutes

Servings: 4

Ingredients:

- 600 g berries (raspberries, blueberries, blackberries)
- 2 small bananas
- 3 tbsp acai powder
- 600 g yogurt alternative made from soy
- 200 ml almond drink (almond milk)
- 2 tbsp light sesame seeds
- 30 g peanuts
- 2 tbsp sunflower seeds
- 2 tbsp pumpkin seeds

Directions:

1. Rinse, sort, and drain the berries; Set aside 50 g each of blueberries and blackberries. Take the bananas out of the peel, break them into pieces and puree them with berries, acai powder, yogurt alternative, and almond

drink to a homogeneous mass. Fill the smoothie into 4 bowls.

2. For draping, roast the sesame seeds with peanuts, sunflower, and pumpkin seeds in a hot pan at a medium temperature.

3. Then set aside for 3 minutes and let cool down. Drape and serve bowls with roasted seeds, nuts and kernels, and the remaining blueberries and blackberries.

Nutrition:

Calories 393

Protein 17 g

Fat 21 g

Carbohydrates 30 g

38. Berry Bowl

Preparation time: 15 minutes

Cooking time: 20 minutes

Servings: 2

Ingredients:

- 100 g quinoa

- 300 ml of milk or water

- 2 handfuls of fruit (strawberries, raspberries, blackberries)

- 2 tbsp peanuts

- Honey to taste

Directions:

1. Wash the quinoa in a sieve with cold water until it runs clear. Bring the milk to a boil and add the quinoa. Cover and simmer at low temperature for about 15 minutes until the grains are soft, stirring occasionally.

2. In the meantime, wash the fruit off, remove the stalk if necessary and cut it into bite-sized pieces. Remove the quinoa from the heat, stir and let rest for another 5 minutes.

3. Divide the finished grain into two bowls, arrange the fruit and peanuts decoratively on top, and drizzle with honey.

Nutrition:

Calories 335

Protein 14 g

Fat 9 g

Carbohydrates 48 g

39. Good Morning Quark

Preparation time: 15 minutes

Cooking time: 0 minutes

Servings: 1

Ingredients:

- 150 g quark (lean)

- 50 g fresh or frozen strawberries

- 30 g blueberries

- 40 g of banana

- 1 teaspoon coconut flakes

- 1 tbsp goji berries

- 1 teaspoon flaxseed

- Agave syrup as needed

Directions:

1. Pour the strawberries and quark into a suitable mixing vessel and puree with the hand blender to a homogeneous mass. Sweeten fruit quark according to personal taste with agave syrup or another sweetener.

2. Wash the blueberries and let them dry. Remove the banana from the skin and cut it into bite-sized slices.

3. Pour the strawberry quark into a bowl and arrange the blueberries, banana slices, linseed, goji berries, and desiccated coconut on top, and serve.

Nutrition:

Calories 235

Protein 21 g

Fat 3 g

Carbohydrates 29 g

40. Apple Porridge

Preparation time: 15 minutes

Cooking time: 10 minutes

Servings: 1

Ingredients:

- 60 g protein porridge
- 1 apple
- 1 tbsp chia seeds
- 1 tbsp crushed flaxseed

Directions:

1. Bring the water to a boil. Pour protein porridge into a bowl with a spoon and pour 120 ml of hot water over it. Stir the porridge well and let it rest for 3 - 5 minutes.

2. In the meantime, wash the apple, cut into four, and remove the core. Finely chop the apple pieces with the grater, then stir into the porridge with the chia and flax seeds and enjoy warm.

Nutrition:

Calories 360

Protein 26 g

Fat 13 g

Carbohydrates 28 g

41. Flakes with Peanuts and Figs

Preparation time: 15 minutes

Cooking time: 0 minutes

Servings: 1

Ingredients:

- 1 peach
- 50 g raspberries
- 1 fig
- 30 g peanuts
- 65 g de-oiled soy flakes
- 250 g soy yogurt

Directions:

1. Put the soy flakes in a bowl. Wash the peach, fig, and raspberries and let them dry. Slice the peach in half, then discard the core from the pulp, then cut into slices. Cut the fig into pieces.

2. Arrange the peach and fig slices with the raspberries on the soy flakes. Add peanuts; you can chop them if you like. Stir in the soy yogurt and mix everything.

Nutrition:

Calories 564

Protein 52 g

Fat 20 g

Carbohydrates 33 g

42. Blueberry Bowl

Preparation time: 15 minutes

Cooking time: 0 minutes

Servings: 1

Ingredients:

- 250 g Greek yogurt
- 1 teaspoon acai powder
- 1 teaspoon cocoa, slightly de-oiled
- 40 g blueberries
- 1 teaspoon chia seeds
- 5 g desiccated coconut
- 1 teaspoon bee pollen
- 1 teaspoon walnuts
- 20 g coconut muesli
- Agave syrup as needed

Directions:

1. Whisk the yogurt with acai powder and cocoa. Sweeten the yogurt to your taste with a little agave syrup, then pour into a bowl.

2. Wash the blueberries and let them dry, then serve on the yogurt. Arrange chia seeds, desiccated coconut, pollen, walnuts, and muesli decoratively on the bowl and serve.

Nutrition:

Calories 545

Protein 17 g

Fat 43 g

Carbohydrates 19 g

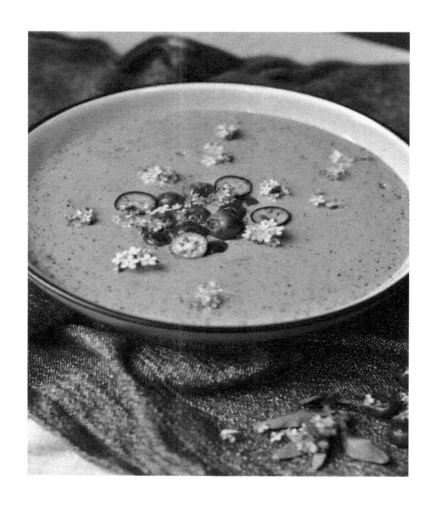

43. Mango and Peanut Breakfast

Preparation time: 15 minutes

Cooking time: 10 minutes

Servings: 1

Ingredients:

- 20 g whole grain oatmeal
- 20 g peanuts chopped
- 2 teaspoons agave syrup
- 1 pinch of cinnamon, ground
- 30 g mango
- 200 ml soy drink, organic

Directions:

1. Roast oatmeal and peanuts in a pan without fat, stir several times in between so that nothing burns. Pour agave syrup and cinnamon into the pan and stir in.

2. Spread the muesli on a large plate to cool. In the meantime, divide the mango pulp into small pieces. Pour muesli with mango and soy drink into a bowl and serve.

Nutrition:

Calories 323

Protein 14 g

Fat 16 g

Carbohydrates 29 g

44. Tofu with Cauliflower

Preparation Time: 5 minutes

Cooking Time: 45 minutes

Servings: 2

Ingredients:

- ¼ cup red pepper, seeded
- 1 Thai chili, cut in two halves, seeded
- 2 cloves of garlic
- 1 tsp of olive oil
- 1 pinch of cumin

- 1 pinch of coriander

- Juice of a half lemon

- 8oz tofu

- 8oz cauliflower, roughly chopped

- 1 ½oz red onions, finely chopped

- 1 tsp finely chopped ginger

- 2 teaspoons turmeric

- 1oz dried tomatoes, finely chopped

- 1oz parsley, chopped

Directions:

1. Preheat oven to 400 °F. Slice the peppers and put them in an ovenproof dish with chili and garlic. Pour some olive oil over it, add the dried herbs, and put it in the oven until the peppers are soft, about 20 minutes.

2. Let it cool down, put the peppers together with the lemon juice in a blender, and work it into a soft mass. Cut the tofu in half and divide the halves into triangles.

3. Place the tofu in a small casserole dish, cover with the paprika mixture, and place in the oven for about 20 minutes. Chop the cauliflower until the pieces are smaller than a grain of rice.

4. Then, in a small saucepan, heat the garlic, onions, chili, and ginger with olive oil until they become transparent.

5. Add turmeric and cauliflower, mix well, and heat again. Remove from heat and add parsley and tomatoes; mix well. Serve with the tofu in the sauce.

Nutrition:

Calories: 248

Carbs: 27g

Fat: 8g

Chapter 2. Mains

45. Sweet and Sour Pan with Cashew Nuts

Preparation Time: 30 minutes

Cooking Time: 0 minutes

Servings: 2

Ingredients:

- 2 tbsp. coconut oil

- 2 red onion

- 2 yellow bell pepper

- 12oz white cabbage

- 6oz Pak choi

- 1 ½ oz mung bean sprouts

- 4 pineapple slices 1 ½ oz cashew nuts

- ¼ cup apple cider vinegar

- 4 tbsp. coconut blossom sugar

- 11/2 tbsp. tomato paste

- 1 tsp coconut-aminos

- 2 tsp arrowroot powder

- ¼ cup of water

Directions:

1. Roughly cut the vegetables. Mix the arrowroot with five tbsp. of cold water into a paste. Put all the other fixing for the sauce in a saucepan and add the arrowroot paste for binding.

2. Dissolve the coconut oil in a pan, then fry the onion. Add the bell pepper, cabbage, Pak choi, and bean sprouts and stir-fry until the vegetables become a little softer.

3. Add the pineapple and cashew nuts and stir a few more times. Pour a little sauce over the wok dish and serve.

Nutrition:

Calories: 65

Carbs: 8g

Fat: 3g

Protein: 1g

46. Fried Cauliflower Rice

Preparation Time: 55 minutes

Cooking Time: 10 minutes

Servings: 2

Ingredients:

- 1 medium cauliflower

- 2 tbsp. coconut oil

- 1 medium red onion

- 4 cloves garlic

- ¼ cup vegetable broth

- 2-inch fresh ginger

- 1 tsp chili flakes

- 1/2 carrot

- 1/2 red bell pepper

- 1/2 lemon, juiced

- 2 tbsp. pumpkin seeds

- 2 tbsp. fresh coriander

Directions:

1. Cut the cauliflower into small rice grains using a food processor. Finely chop the onion, garlic, and ginger, cut the carrot into thin strips, dice the bell pepper and finely chop the herbs.

2. Melt 1 tbsp of coconut oil in a pan and add half of the onion and garlic to the pan and fry briefly until translucent. Add cauliflower rice and season with salt.

3. Pour in the broth and stir everything until it evaporates and the cauliflower rice is tender. Take the rice out of the pan and set it aside.

4. Melt the rest of the coconut oil in the pan and add the remaining onions, garlic, ginger, carrots, and peppers. Fry for a few minutes until the vegetables are tender. Season them with a little salt. Serve.

Nutrition:

Calories: 289

Carbs: 11g

Fat: 9g

Protein: 31g

47. Buckwheat with Onions

Preparation Time: 10 minutes

Cooking Time: 40 minutes

Servings: 4

Ingredients:

- 3 cups of buckwheat, rinsed
- 4 medium red onions, chopped
- 1 big white onion, chopped
- 5 oz. extra-virgin olive oil
- 3 cups of water
- Salt and pepper, to taste

Directions:

1. Dip and soak the buckwheat in the warm water within 10 minutes. Then add the buckwheat to your pot. Add in the water, salt, and pepper to your pot and stir well. Close the lid and cook for about 30-35 minutes until the buckwheat is ready.

2. In the meantime, in a skillet, heat the extra-virgin olive oil and fry the chopped onions for 15 minutes until clear and caramelized.

3. Add some salt and pepper and mix well. Portion the buckwheat into four bowls or mugs. Then dollop each bowl with the onions. Remember that this dish should be served warm.

Nutrition:

Calories: 154

Carbs: 33g

Fat: 1g

Protein: 6g

48. Dahl with Kale, Red Onions, and Buckwheat

Preparation time: 5 minutes

Cooking time: 20 minutes

Servings: 2

Ingredients:

- 1 tsp. of extra virgin olive oil

- 1 tsp. of mustard seeds

- 1 ½ oz. red onions, finely chopped

- 1 clove of garlic, very finely chopped

- 1 tsp very finely chopped ginger

- 1 Thai chili, very finely chopped

- 1 tsp. curry powder

- 2 tsp. turmeric

- 10 fl. oz. vegetable broth

- 1 ½ oz. red lentils

- 1 5/8 oz. kale, chopped

- 1.70 fl. oz. coconut milk

- 1 5/8 oz. buckwheat

Directions:

1. Heat oil in a pan at medium temperature and add mustard seeds. When they crack, add onion, garlic, ginger, and chili. Heat until everything is soft.

2. Add the curry powder and turmeric, mix well. Add the vegetable stock, bring to the boil, then put the lentils and cook them for 25 to 30 minutes until they are ready.

3. Then add the kale and coconut milk and simmer for 5 minutes. The dahl is ready. While the lentils are cooking, prepare the buckwheat. Serve buckwheat with the dahl.

Nutrition:

Calories: 151

Carbs: 0g

Fat: 0g

Protein: 0g

49. Miso Caramelized Tofu

Preparation Time: 55 minutes

Cooking Time: 15 minutes

Servings: 2

Ingredients:

- 1 tbsp mirin
- ¾ oz. miso paste
- 5 ¼ oz. firm tofu
- 1 ½ oz. celery, trimmed
- 1 ¼ oz. red onion
- 4 ¼ oz. zucchini
- 1 bird's eye chili
- 1 garlic clove, finely chopped
- 1 tsp. fresh ginger, finely chopped
- 1 5/8 oz. kale, chopped
- 2 tsp. sesame seeds
- 1 ¼ oz. buckwheat
- 1 tsp. ground turmeric
- 2 tsp. extra virgin olive oil

- 1 tsp. tamari (or soy sauce)

Directions

1. Preheat your over to 400°F. Cover a tray with parchment paper. Combine the mirin and miso. Dice the tofu and let marinate it in the mirin-miso mixture.

2. Chop the vegetables (except for the kale) at a diagonal angle to produce long slices. Using a steamer, cook the kale for 5 minutes and set aside.

3. Disperse the tofu across the lined tray and garnish with sesame seeds. Roast for 20 minutes, or until caramelized. Rinse the buckwheat using running water and a sieve.

4. Add to a pan of boiling water alongside turmeric and cook the buckwheat according to the packet instructions. Heat the oil in a skillet over high heat.

5. Toss in the vegetables, herbs, and spices, then fry for 2-3 minutes. Adjust to medium heat and fry for a further 5 minutes or until cooked but still crunchy.

Nutrition:

Calories: 34

Carbs: 3g

Fat: 1g

Protein: 1g

50. Miso Caramelized Tofu

Preparation Time: 20 minutes

Cooking Time: 30 minutes

Servings: 4

Ingredients:

- 1 cup cooked cannellini beans
- 8 oz. tempeh
- ¼ cup cooked bulgur
- 2 cloves garlic, pressed
- ¼ tsp onion powder
- 1 tsp liquid smoke
- 4 tsp Worcestershire sauce
- 1 tsp smoked paprika
- 2 tbsp. organic ketchup
- 2 tbsp. maple syrup
- 2 tbsp. neutral-flavored oil
- 3 tbsp. tamari
- ¼ cup chickpea flour
- Nonstick cooking spray

Directions:

1. Mash the beans in a large bowl. Crumble the tempeh into small pieces on top. Add the bulgur and garlic.

2. In a medium bowl, whisk the remaining ingredients, except the flour and cooking spray. Stir into the crumbled tempeh preparation. Add the flour and mix until well combined. Chill for 1 hour before shaping into patties.

3. Preheat the oven to 350°F. Line a baking tray with parchment paper. Scoop out 1/3 cup per patty, shaping into an approximately 3-inch circle and flattening slightly on the tray.

4. Lightly coat the top of the patties with cooking spray. Bake for 15 minutes, carefully flip, and lightly coat the top of the patties with cooking spray and bake for another 15 minutes until lightly browned and firm. Serve.

Nutrition:

Calories: 120

Carbs: 9g

Fat: 7g

Protein: 7g

51. Tomato & Goat's Cheese Pizza

Preparation Time: 5 Minutes + 2 hours

Cooking Time: 50 Minutes

Servings: 2

Ingredients:

- 8oz buckwheat flour
- 2 tsp. dried yeast
- Pinch of salt
- 5fl oz. slightly water
- 1 tsp. olive oil
- 3oz feta cheese, crumbled
- 3oz passata or tomato paste
- 1 tomato, sliced
- 1 medium red onion, finely chopped
- 1oz arugula leaves, chopped

Directions:

1. Mix all the fixing for the pizza dough and stand for at least two hours until it has doubled in size in a bowl.

2. Roll the dough out to a size to suit you. Spoon the passata onto the base and add the rest of the toppings.

Bake in the oven at 400F within 15-20 minutes or until browned at the edges and crispy and serve.

Nutrition:

Calories: 180

Carbs: 21g

Fat: 6g

Protein: 10g

52. Green Beans with Crispy Chickpeas

Preparation Time: 30 minutes

Cooking Time: 10 minutes

Servings: 4

Ingredients:

- 1 can chickpeas, rinsed

- 1 tsp. whole coriander

- 1 lb. green beans, trimmed

- 2 tbsp. olive oil, divided

- Kosher salt and freshly ground black pepper

- 1 tsp. cumin seeds

- Grilled lemons for serving

Directions

1. Heat grill to medium. Gather chickpeas, coriander, cumin, and 1 tbsp oil in a medium cast-iron skillet.

2. Put the skillet on the grill and cook chickpeas, occasionally mixing, until golden brown and coriander begin to pop, 5 to 6 minutes. Season with salt and pepper.

3. Transfer to a bowl. Add green beans and remaining tbsp of olive oil to the skillet. Add salt and pepper.

4. Cook, turning once, until charred and barely tender, 3 to 4 minutes. Toss green beans with chickpea mixture and serve with grilled lemons alongside.

Nutrition:

Calories: 59

Carbs: 11g

Fat: 1g

Protein: 2g

53. Baked Potatoes with Spicy Chickpea Stew

Preparation Time: 10 minutes

Cooking Time: 60 minutes

Servings: 4

Ingredients:

- 4 baking potatoes, pricked around
- 2 tbsp. olive oil
- 2 red onions, finely chopped
- 4 tsp. garlic, crushed or grated
- 1-inch ginger, grated
- 1/2 tsp chili flakes
- 2 tbsp. cumin seeds
- 2 tbsp. turmeric
- Splash of water
- 2 tins chopped tomatoes
- 2 tbsp. cocoa powder, unsweetened
- 2 tins chickpeas – do not drain
- 2 yellow peppers, chopped

Directions:

1. Preheat the oven to 400F, and start preparing all ingredients. When the oven is ready, put in baking potatoes and cook for 50 minutes-1 hours until they are done.

2. While potatoes are cooking, put olive oil and sliced red onion into a large wide saucepan and cook lightly, using the lid, for 5 minutes until the onions are tender but not brown.

3. Remove the lid and add ginger, garlic, cumin, and cook for a further minute on low heat. Then add the turmeric and a tiny dab of water and cook for a few more minutes.

4. Then add tomatoes, cocoa powder, peppers, chickpeas with their water and salt. Boil, and then simmer on low heat within 45-50 minutes until it's thick.

5. Finally, stir in the 2 tbsp of parsley, some pepper, salt if you desire, and serve the stew with the potatoes.

Nutrition:

Calories: 392

Carbs: 80g

Fat: 6g

Protein: 12g

54. Broccoli and Pasta

Preparation Time: 20 minutes

Cooking Time: 10 minutes

Servings: 2

Ingredients:

- 5 oz. spaghetti

- 5 oz. broccoli

- 1 garlic clove, finely chopped

- 3 tbsp. extra virgin olive oil

- 2 Shallots sliced

- ¼ tsp. crushed chilies

- 12 sage shredded leaves

- Grated parmesan (optional)

Directions:

1. Put broccoli in boiling water within 5 minutes, then add spaghetti and cook until both pasta and broccoli are done (around 8 to 10 minutes).

2. In the meantime, warm oil in a frying pan and add shallots and garlic. Cook for 5 minutes until it becomes golden. Mix chilies and sage to the pan and gently cook for more than 1 minute.

3. Drain pasta and broccoli; mix with the shallot mixture in the pan; add some Parmesan, if desired, and serve.

Nutrition:

Calories: 150

Carbs: 17g

Fat: 8g

Protein: 6g

55. Artichokes and Kale with Walnuts

Preparation Time: 10 minutes

Cooking Time: 30 minutes

Servings: 2

Ingredients:

- 1 cup of artichoke hearts
- 1 tbsp. parsley, chopped
- ½ cup of walnuts
- 1 cup of kale, torn
- 1 cup of Cheddar cheese, crumbled
- ½ tbsp. balsamic vinegar
- 1 tbsp. olive oil
- Salt and black pepper, to taste

Directions:

1. Preheat the oven to 250-270 F and roast the walnuts in the oven for 10 minutes until lightly browned and crispy, and then set aside.

2. Add artichoke hearts, kale, oil, salt, and pepper to a pot and cook for 20-25 minutes until done. Add cheese and balsamic vinegar and stir well. Divide the vegetables

into two plates and garnish with roasted walnuts and parsley.

Nutrition:

Calories: 100

Carbs: 12g

Fat: 4g

Protein: 4g

56. Grilled Veggie Kabobs

Preparation time: 15 minutes

Cooking time:

12-15 minutes

Servings: 6

Ingredients:

Marinade:

- ½ cup balsamic vinegar

- 1½ tablespoons minced thyme

- 1½ tablespoons minced rosemary

- 3 cloves garlic, peeled and minced

- Sea salt, to taste (optional)

- Freshly ground black pepper, to taste

Veggies:

- 2 cups cherry tomatoes

- 1 red bell pepper should be seeded and cut into 1-inch pieces

- 1 green bell pepper, without seeds and cut into 1-inch pieces

- 1 medium yellow squash, cut into 1-inch rounds

- 1 medium zucchini, cut into 1-inch rounds

- 1 medium red onion skinned and cut into large chunks

Special Equipment:

- 12 bamboo skewers, make sure to soak it in water for 30 minutes

Directions:

1. Preheat the grill to medium heat.

2. For the marinade, stir the balsamic vinegar, thyme, rosemary, garlic, salt (if desired), and pepper in a small bowl. Thread veggies onto skewers, alternating between different-colored veggies.

3. Grill the veggies for 12 to 15 minutes until softened and lightly charred, brushing the veggies with the marinade and flipping the skewers every 4 to 5 minutes. Remove from the grill and serve hot.

Nutrition:

Calories: 98

Fat: 0.7g

Carbs: 19.2g

Protein: 3.8g

57. Grilled Cauliflower Steaks

Preparation Time: 10 Minutes

Cooking Time: 57 Minutes

Servings: 4

Ingredients:

- 2 medium heads cauliflower
- 2 medium shallots, peeled and minced
- Water, as needed
- 1 clove garlic, peeled and minced
- ½ teaspoon ground fennel
- ½ teaspoon minced sage
- ½ teaspoon crushed red pepper flakes
- ½ cup green lentils, rinsed
- 2 cups low-sodium vegetable broth
- Salt, to taste (optional)
- Freshly ground black pepper, to taste
- Chopped parsley, for garnish

Directions:

1. On a flat work surface, cut each of the cauliflower heads in half through the stem, then trim each half, so you get a 1-inch-thick steak. Arrange each piece on a baking sheet and set aside. You can reserve the extra cauliflower florets for other uses.

2. Sauté the shallots in a medium saucepan over medium heat for 10 minutes, stirring occasionally. Add water, 1 to 3 tablespoons at a time, to keep the shallots from sticking.

3. Stir in the garlic, fennel, sage, red pepper flakes, and lentils and cook for 3 minutes. Pour into the vegetable broth and bring to a boil over high heat. Reduce the heat to medium, cover, and cook for 45 to 50 minutes, or until the lentils are very soft, adding more water as needed.

4. Using an immersion blender, purée the mixture until smooth. Sprinkle with salt (if desired) and pepper. Keep warm and set aside.

5. Preheat the grill to medium heat. Grill the cauliflower steaks for about 7 minutes per side until evenly browned. Transfer the cauliflower steaks to a plate and spoon the purée over them. Serve garnished with the parsley.

Nutrition:

Calories: 105

Fat: 1.1g

Carbs: 18.3g

Protein: 5.4g

58. Vegetable Hash with White Beans

Preparation time: 15 minutes

Cooking time:

23 minutes

Servings: 4

Ingredients:

- 1 leek (white part only), finely chopped
- 1 red bell pepper, deseeded and diced
- Water, as needed
- 2 teaspoons minced rosemary
- 3 cloves garlic, peeled and minced
- 1 medium sweet potato, peeled and diced
- 1 large turnip, peeled and diced
- 2 cups cooked white beans
- Zest and juice of 1 orange
- 1 cup chopped kale
- Salt, to taste (optional)
- Freshly ground black pepper, to taste

Directions:

1. Put the leek and red pepper in a large saucepan over medium heat and sauté for 8 minutes, stirring occasionally. Add water, 1 to 3 tablespoons at a time, to keep them from sticking to the bottom of the pan.

2. Stir in the rosemary and garlic and sauté for 1 minute more. Add the sweet potato, turnip, beans, and orange juice and zest, and stir well—heat until the vegetables are softened.

3. Add the kale and sprinkle with salt (if desired) and pepper. Cook for about 5 minutes or more until the kale is wilted. Serve on a plate.

Nutrition:

Calories: 245

Fat: 0.6g

Carbs: 48.0g

Protein: 11.9g

59. Green Tagliatelle with Pistachio Gremolata

Preparation Time: 10 minutes

Cooking Time: 30 minutes

Servings: 2

Ingredients:

- 1 organic juice orange

- 1 tablespoon pistachio, roasted, chopped

- garlic, chopped

- 0.5 tbsp thyme leaves, chopped

- 1 tablespoon chopped parsley

- pepper, freshly ground

- 50 grams green soybean pasta

- salt

- 10 grams of green bell pepper, halved lengthways, cored

- 3rd spring onions, in rings

- 1 tablespoon of olive oil

- 1 tomato, chopped

- 1 tablespoon balsamic vinegar, white

- 1tablespoons chili sauce, sweet and spicy

Directions:

1. For the pistachio gremolata, rinse the orange hot, dry, and grate 1 tbsp orange peel. Mix with the pistachios, garlic, thyme, and parsley. Season the gremolata vigorously with pepper. Squeeze the orange to juice and set aside.

2. Cook the noodles in salted water, braise onions and green peppers in olive oil. Add tomatoes and melt briefly.

3. Put salt and pepper, then orange juice and vinegar, and boil. Drain the noodles, mix with peppers and chili sauce and serve with the gremolata.

Nutrition:

Calories: 214

Protein: 7.13 g

Fat: 9.19 g

Carbohydrates: 31.21 g

60. Zucchini and Bean Salad with Spinach Flan

Preparation Time:10 minutes

Cooking Time: 35 minutes

Servings: 3

Ingredients:

- cooked spinach flans

- 150 grams of legumes

- 150 grams of zucchini, in fine strips

- salt

- 6 tablespoons of lemon juice

- 1 tablespoon of balsamic vinegar

- 1 clove of garlic, chopped

- 1 tablespoon acacia honey, liquid

- pepper, freshly ground

- 2 tablespoons of olive oil

- 2 tsp linseed oil

- 1 red onion, in fine rings

- 2 sticks of celery, in thin slices

- 1 handful of mint, fresh leaves

Directions:

1. Prepare frozen legumes, drain, and let cool. Salt the zucchini strips a little. Mix the lemon juice, vinegar, garlic, honey, and pepper. Fold in olive oil and linseed oil with a fork.

2. Mix legume mix, onion, celery, zucchini with liquid, mint, and vinaigrette and arrange with both spinach flans on deep plates or bowls.

Nutrition:

Calories: 276

Protein: 15.83 g

Fat: 14.34 g

Carbohydrates: 31.06 g

61. Papaya Bowl

Preparation Time: 0 minutes

Cooking Time: 15minutes

Servings: 2

Ingredients:

- 40 grams of iceberg lettuce, cut
- 140 grams of papaya, papaya pulp, sliced
- 1 tbsp papaya seeds
- 50 grams of cucumber, sliced
- 1/2 red peppers, finely sliced
- 2 tablespoons of lime juice
- 1 tsp camelina oil
- pepper, freshly ground
- salt
- 40 grams of bread

Directions:

1. Fill iceberg lettuce, papaya, papaya seeds, cucumber, and bell pepper into a storage box or lunch box.

2. Mix lime juice, camelina oil, pepper, salt, and 1-2 teaspoons of water and drizzle over the vegetables. Close the can. Pack the bread strips separately.

Nutrition:

Calories: 646

Protein: 30.46 g

Fat: 10.45 g

Carbohydrates: 114.11 g

62. Spicy Muesli with Sheep's Cheese

Preparation Time:10 minutes

Cooking Time: 10 minutes

Servings: 2

Ingredients:

- 150 grams of kefir
- 1 tsp tomato paste
- 1 tablespoon acacia honey or rosemary honey
- 1 tsp soy sauce
- cayenne pepper
- 50 grams of sheep's cheese
- Cucumber, in cubes
- 1 kiwi, gold kiwi, sliced
- 3 tablespoons of muesli

Directions:

1. Mix the kefir, tomato paste, honey, and soy sauce and season with cayenne pepper. Roughly crumble sheep's cheese. Put kefir, cucumber, kiwi, and sheep's cheese in a transport container and sprinkle with muesli.

Nutrition:

Calories: 487

Protein: 39.81 g

Fat: 7.61 g

Carbohydrates: 138.19 g

63. Pumpernickel Sandwich

Preparation Time: 10 minutes

Cooking Time: 10 minutes

Servings: 2

Ingredients:

- 60 grams of sour milk cheese

- pepper, freshly ground

- 2 pumpernickel slices (80 g)

- 1 tablespoon of tomato paste

- 40 grams of arugula

- 2 pickled gherkins (sliced)

- 1 apple (half in thin slices, half whole)

- 1 teaspoon of lemon juice

- 1 tsp mustard (sweet)

Directions:

1. Cut the cheese into four pieces and pepper. Spread a tomato paste on the slice of bread and top with arugula, cheese, and pickled cucumbers.

2. Drizzle lemon slices and the whole half of the cut surface with lemon juice. Spread the slices over the cucumbers. Brush the other slice of bread with mustard and cover the apple slices. Serve.

Nutrition:

Calories: 270

Protein: 36.76 g

Fat: 10.12 g

Carbohydrates: 10.47 g

64. Hazelnut Porridge with Pear

Preparation Time: 10 minutes

Cooking Time: 5 minutes

Servings: 2

Ingredients:

- 1 tsp camelina oil
- 1 tbsp maple syrup
- 2 knife sp. cardamom (ground)
- 3 tablespoons of orange juice
- 3 tablespoons of oatmeal
- salt
- 1 tablespoon flaxseed
- 150 grams of pear (in columns)
- 3 tablespoons hazelnut leaves (roasted)
- 1 passion fruit (passion fruit)

Directions:

1. Mix the camelina oil, maple syrup, cardamom, and orange juice. Boil 150 ml of water. Add oatmeal, a pinch of salt, and flaxseed and cook everything with a whisk for 2-3 minutes. Arrange porridge with pears,

hazelnuts, the juicy seeds of the passion fruit, and orange syrup.

Nutrition:

Calories: 356

Protein: 15.46 g

Fat: 18.45 g

Carbohydrates: 74.11 g

65. Porridge with Pineapple

Preparation Time:10 minutes

Cooking Time: 10 minutes

Servings: 2

Ingredients:

- 70 ml of oat milk

- 2 pinch of turmeric (ground)

- 2 pinch of coriander (ground)

- 40 grams of millet (millet-buckwheat porridge, or oatmeal)

- 100 grams of pineapple (in cubes)

- 1 tsp rapeseed oil

- 50 grams of frozen blueberries

- 1 tsp ginger syrup

- 2 tbsp walnuts (chopped)

Directions:

1. Boil 50 ml water, oat drink, spices, and millet-buckwheat mixture according to the package instructions.

2. Roast the pineapple cubes in rapeseed oil. Add blueberries, ginger syrup, walnuts, arrange the porridge with the fruits.

Nutrition:

Calories: 138

Protein: 3.79 g

Fat: 13.77

Carbohydrates: 1.85 g

66. Flax Seed Curd with Apple and Cucumber

Preparation Time:10 minutes

Cooking Time: 0 minutes

Servings: 4

Ingredients:

- 150 grams of herb curd
- 150 grams of cream cheese
- 1 tablespoon linseed oil
- 3 tablespoons of lemon juice
- 2 tablespoons flaxseed, crushed
- seasoned salt
- pepper, freshly ground
- 3 tablespoons chives, rolls, fresh or frozen
- 1 apple
- 1 mini cucumber
- linseed
- chives (for sprinkling)

Directions:

1. Mix the herb curd, linseed oil, lemon juice, linseed, cream cheese, and season with herb salt and pepper. Stir in chives.

2. Rinse the apple and cucumber hot and grate dry. Quarter the apple, core it, and cut it into thick slices, cucumber into long sticks. Arrange the quark, apple, and cucumber and sprinkle with flax seeds and chives.

Nutrition:

Calories: 100

Protein: 1.89 g

Fat: 5.8 g

Carbohydrates: 12.45 g

67. Bread Topped with Egg and Mustard Cream

Preparation Time: 10 minutes

Cooking Time: 15 minutes

Servings: 2

Ingredients:

- 1 tbsp mustard, sweet
- 2 tsp mustard, spicy
- 2 tablespoons of orange juice
- 2 el low-fat curd
- 1 teaspoon quark
- 1 tablespoons chive, rolls, fresh or frozen
- Pepper, freshly ground
- salt
- 1 slice of bread
- 1/2 handful of lettuce
- 40 grams of pickled onion, sliced
- 1 organic egg, hard-boiled

Directions:

1. Mix both mustard, orange juice, 2 tbsp curd cheese, and chives and season the cream with pepper and salt.

2. Spread 1 teaspoon of curd on the bread slice, add the salad on a plate, and onions. Pour a dollop of mustard cream over it, arrange the remaining cream, and the halved egg.

Nutrition:

Calories: 198

Protein: 5.33 g

Fat: 13.51 g

Carbohydrates: 11.82 g

Chapter 3. Side

68. Nutty Green Beans

Preparation time: 10 minutes

Cooking time: 5 minutes

Servings: 2

Ingredients:

- 2 tbsp. each chunky-style peanut butter

- 2 tbsp sherry

- 2 tsp. oyster sauce

- 1 garlic clove, minced

- 1/2 tsp. minced pared ginger root

- 2 cups cooked frozen French-style green beans (hot)

Directions:

1. In a small saucepan, combine peanut butter, sherry, oyster sauce, garlic, and ginger; bring to a boil. Reduce heat and let simmer, continually stirring until the mixture is creamy, about 1 minute. Pour peanut butter mixture over hot green beans and serve immediately.

Nutrition:

Calories 157

Fat 8 g

Carbs 3 g

Protein 7 g

69. Vegetable-Cottage Cheese

70. Grilled Asparagus with Caper Vinaigrette

Preparation time: 10 minutes

Cooking time: 5 minutes

Servings: 6

Ingredients:

- 1 ½ lb. asparagus spears, trimmed
- 2 tsp. caper, coarsely chopped
- 1 tbsp. red wine vinegar
- 1 garlic clove, minced
- 3 tbsp. Extra virgin olive oil
- ¼ cup small basil leaves
- ½ tsp. Dijon mustard
- Cooking spray
- ½ tsp. Kosher salt, divided
- ¼ tsp. ground black pepper

Directions:

1. Preheat grill to medium-high heat. Place asparagus in a shallow dish. Add 1 tbsp oil and ¼ tsp, and salt, tossing well to coat. Place asparagus on grill rack coated with cooking spray.

2. Grill 4 minutes or until crisp-tender, turning after 2 minutes. Combine remaining ¼ tsp: salt, vinegar, mustard, and garlic.

3. Stir with a whisk. Slowly pour the remaining 2 tbsp of oil into the vinegar mixture, continually stirring with a whisk. Stir in capers. Arrange asparagus on a serving platter. Drizzle with vinaigrette and sprinkle with basil.

Nutrition:

Calories 89

Fat 6.9g

Carbs 4.7g

Protein 2.8g

71.Cheesy Asparagus

Preparation time: 10 minutes

Cooking time: 15 minutes

Servings: 4

Ingredients:

- 1 lb. asparagus, trimmed
- 2 tbsp. olive oil
- ½ cup Parmesan cheese, shredded
- ½ cup mozzarella cheese, shredded
- 1 tbsp. Italian seasoning
- Black pepper and sea salt to taste:

Directions:

1. Warm oven to 400° F. Line a baking sheet with foil or parchment paper. Mix the asparagus with olive oil, sea

salt, black pepper, plus half of the Italian seasoning.

2. Put in a single layer on the lined baking sheet. Roast in the oven for about 8 minutes, until the asparagus is bright green and just starting to soften.

3. Mix the mozzarella plus Parmesan cheese, then sprinkle over the asparagus. Top with remaining Italian seasoning. Return to the oven within 7 minutes, until the cheese is melted and golden.

Nutrition:

Calories 160

Fat 12g

Carbs 3g

Protein 8g

72. Stuffed Avocado

Preparation time: 10 minutes

Cooking time: 0 minutes

Servings: 2

Ingredients:

- 2 tbsp. light mayonnaise

- 1 tsp. chopped fresh chives

- ¼ cup peeled and diced cucumber

- 2 tsp. sriracha, plus more for drizzling

- 1 small avocado (pitted and peeled)

- ½ tsp. furikake

- 2 tsp. gluten-free soy sauce

Directions:

1. Mix mayonnaise, sriracha, and chives in a medium bowl. Add cucumber, plus chive, and gently toss. Cut the avocado open, remove the pit and peel the skin or spoon the avocado out. Fill the avocado halves equally with crab salad. Top with furikake and drizzle with soy sauce.

Nutrition:

Calories 194

Fat 13g

Carbs 7g

Protein 12g

73. Kale Sauté

Preparation time: 10 minutes

Cooking time: 15 minutes

Servings: 2

Ingredients:

- 1 chopped red onion
- 3 tbsps. coconut aminos
- 2 tbsps. olive oil
- 1 lb. torn kale
- 1 tbsp. chopped cilantro
- 1 tbsp. lime juice
- 2 minced garlic cloves

Directions:

1. Heat-up a pan with the olive oil over medium heat, add the onion and the garlic, and sauté for 5 minutes. Add the kale and the other ingredients, toss, cook over medium heat for 10 minutes, divide between plates and serve.

Nutrition:

Calories 200

Fat 7.1 g

Carbs 6.4 g

Protein 6 g

74. Garlic Hummus

Preparation time: 5 minutes

Cooking time: 10 minutes

Servings: 4

Ingredients:

- 3 tbsp freshly squeezed lemon juice
- all- purpose salt-free seasoning
- 3 tbsps. sesame tahini
- 4 garlic cloves
- 15 oz. no-salt-added garbanzo beans, rinsed & drained
- 2 tbsps. olive oil

Directions:

1. Place all the fixing in a food processor, then pulse until smooth. Serve immediately.

Nutrition:

Calories 103

Fat 5 g

Carbs 11 g

Protein 4 g

75. Sage Carrots

Preparation Time: 10 minutes

Cooking Time: 30 minutes

Servings: 2

Ingredients:

- 2 tsp sweet paprika
- 1 tbsp chopped sage
- 2 tbsp olive oil
- 1 lb. peeled and roughly cubed carrots
- ¼ tsp black pepper
- 1 chopped red onion

Directions:

1. In a baking pan, combine the carrots with the oil and the other ingredients, toss and bake at 380 0F for 30 minutes.

Divide between plates and serve.

Nutrition:

Calories: 200

Fat: 8.7 g

Carbs: 7.9 g

Protein: 4 g

76. Minty Tomatoes and Corn

Preparation Time: 10 minutes

Cooking Time: 65 minutes

Servings: 2

Ingredients:

- 2 cups corn
- 1 tbsp rosemary vinegar
- 2 tbsp chopped mint
- 1 lb. sliced tomatoes
- ¼ tsp black pepper
- 2 tbsp olive oil

Directions:

1. In a salad bowl, combine the tomatoes with the corn and the other ingredients, toss and serve. Enjoy!

Nutrition:

Calories: 230

Fat: 7.2 g

Carbs: 11.6 g/Protein: 4g

77 . Roasted Beets

Preparation Time: 10 minutes

Cooking Time: 30 minutes

Servings: 2

Ingredients:

- 2 minced garlic cloves
- ¼ tsp black pepper
- 4 peeled and sliced beets
- ¼ cup chopped walnuts
- 2 tbsp olive oil
- ¼ cup chopped parsley

Directions:

1. Mix the beets with the oil and the other ingredients in a baking dish, toss to coat, put in the oven at 420°F, and bake for 30 minutes. Divide between plates and serve.

Nutrition:

Calories: 156

Fat: 11.8 g

Carbs: 11.5 g

Protein: 3.8 g

78.Rosemary Endives

Preparation Time: 10 minutes

Cooking Time: 20 minutes

Servings: 2

Ingredients:

- 2 tbsp olive oil
- 1 tsp dried rosemary
- 2 halved endives
- ¼ tsp black pepper
- ½ tsp turmeric powder

Directions:

1. In a baking pan, combine the endives with the oil and the other ingredients, toss gently, introduce in the oven and bake at 400 0F for 20 minutes. Divide between plates and serve.

Nutrition:

Calories: 66

Fat: 7.1 g

Carbs: 1.2 g

Protein: 0.3 g

79. Thyme Mushrooms

Preparation Time: 10 minutes

Cooking Time: 30 minutes

Servings: 2

Ingredients:

- 1 tbsp chopped thyme
- 2 tbsp olive oil
- 2 tbsp chopped parsley
- 4 minced garlic cloves
- salt and black pepper to taste
- 2 lbs. halved white mushrooms

Directions:

1. In a baking pan, combine the mushrooms with the garlic and the other ingredients, toss, introduce in the oven and cook at 400°F for 30 minutes. Divide between plates and serve.

Nutrition:

Calories: 251

Fat: 9.3 g

Carbs: 13.2 g

Protein: 6 g

80. Apples and Cabbage Mix

Preparation Time: 10 minutes

Cooking Time:

Servings: 4

Ingredients:

- 2 cored and cubed green apples

- 2 tbsp balsamic vinegar

- ½ tsp caraway seeds

- 2 tbsp olive oil

- black pepper

- 1 shredded red cabbage head

Directions:

1. Mix the cabbage with the apples and the other ingredients in a bowl, toss and serve.

Nutrition:

Calories: 165

Fat: 7.4 g

Carbs: 26 g Protein: 2.6 g

81.Carrot, Tomato, And Arugula Quinoa Pilaf

Preparation Time: 10 minutes

Cooking Time: 22 minutes

Servings: 4

Ingredients:

- 2 teaspoons extra virgin olive oil
- ½ red onion, chopped
- 1 cup quinoa, raw
- 2 cups vegetable or chicken broth
- 1 tsp fresh lovage, chopped
- 1 carrot, chopped
- 1 tomato, chopped
- 1 cup baby arugula

Directions:

1. Heat-up olive oil in a saucepan over medium heat and add the red onion. Cook and stir until translucent, about 5 minutes.

2. Lower the heat, stir in quinoa, and toast, continually stirring, for 2 minutes. Stir in the broth, black pepper, and thyme.

3. Raise the heat to be high and bring it to a boil. Cover, adjust to low and simmer for 5 minutes. Stir in the carrots, cover, and simmer until all water is absorbed about 10 more minutes.

4. Turn off the heat, add tomatoes, arugula and lovage and let sit for 5 minutes. Add salt and pepper to taste.

Nutrition:

Calories: 165

Fat: 4g

Carbs: 27g

Protein: 6g

82. Bake Kale Walnut

Preparation Time: 10 minutes

Cooking Time: 30 minutes

Servings: 4

Ingredients:

- 1 medium red onion, finely chopped
- ¼ cup extra virgin olive oil
- 2 cups baby kale
- ½ cup half-and-half cream
- ½ cup walnuts, coarsely chopped
- 1/3 cup dry breadcrumbs
- ½ tsp ground nutmeg
- Salt and pepper to taste
- ¼ cup dry breadcrumbs
- 2 tbsp. extra virgin olive oil

Directions:

1. Warm oven to 350 degrees F. In a skillet, sauté onion in olive oil until tender. In a large bowl, combine cooked onion, kale, cream, walnuts, breadcrumbs, nutmeg, salt, and pepper to taste, mixing well.

2. Transfer to a greased 1-1/2-qt—baking dish. Combine topping ingredients and sprinkle over the kale mixture. Bake, uncovered, within 30 minutes or until lightly browned.

Nutrition:

Calories: 555

Fat: 31g

Carbs: 65g

Protein: 26g

83. Arugula with Apples and Pine Nuts

Preparation Time: 10 minutes

Cooking Time: 8 minutes

Servings: 4

Ingredients:

- 2 tbsp extra virgin olive oil

- 2 cloves garlic, slivered

- 2 tbsp pine nuts

- 1 apple, peeled, cored, and chopped

- 10 oz. arugula

- Salt and pepper to taste

Directions:

1. Warm-up olive oil in a large skillet or wok over low heat. Put the garlic, pine nuts, and apple. Cook within 3 to 5 minutes.

2. Adjust the heat to medium and add the arugula. Stir and cook another 2 to 3 minutes — season with salt and pepper to taste.

Nutrition:

Calories: 121

Fat: 9g

Carbs: 8g

Protein: 3g

84. Kale Green Bean Casserole

Preparation Time: 5 minutes

Cooking Time: 40 minutes

Servings: 4

Ingredients:

- 1 ½ cups milk
- 1 cup sour cream
- 1 cup mushrooms, chopped
- 2 cups green beans, chopped
- 2 cups kale, chopped
- ¼ cup capers, drained
- ¼ cup walnuts, crushed

Directions:

1. Warm oven to 375 degrees F and lightly greases a casserole dish. Whisk the milk and sour cream together in a large bowl.

2. Add mushrooms, green beans, kale, and capers. Pour into the casserole dish and top with the crushed walnuts. Bake uncovered in the preheated oven until bubbly and browned on top, about 40 minutes.

Nutrition:

Calories: 130

Fat: 6g

Carbs: 14g

Protein: 2g

85.Rice with Lemon and Arugula

Preparation Time: 10 minutes

Cooking Time: 35 minutes

Servings: 4

Ingredients:

- 1 small red onion, chopped
- 1 cup fresh mushrooms, sliced
- 2 cloves garlic, minced
- 1 tbsp. extra-virgin olive oil
- 3 cups long-grain rice, steamed
- 10 oz. fresh arugula
- 3 tbsp. lemon juice
- ¼ tsp dill weed
- Salt and pepper to taste
- 1/3 cup feta cheese, crumbled

Directions:

1. Preheat an oven to 350°F. In a skillet, sauté the onion, mushrooms, and garlic in oil until tender. Stir in the rice, arugula, lemon juice, dill, and salt and pepper to taste.

2. Reserve 1 tbsp cheese and stir the rest into skillet; mix well. Transfer to an 8-in. square baking dish coated with nonstick cooking spray. Sprinkle with reserved cheese.

3. Cover and bake for 25 minutes. Uncover and bake for an additional 5-10 minutes or until heated through, and cheese is melted.

Nutrition:

Calories 290

Fat 6g

Carbohydrate 55g

Protein 13g

86. Cajun Grilled Veggies

Preparation Time: 50 minutes

Cooking Time: 5 minutes

Servings: 4

Ingredients:

- ¼ cup extra virgin olive oil
- 1 tsp Cajun seasoning
- 1/2 tsp cayenne pepper
- 1 tbsp. Worcestershire sauce
- 2 zucchinis cut into 1/2-inch slices
- 2 large red onions, sliced into ½" wedges
- 2 yellow squash, slice into 1/2-inch slices

Directions:

1. Mix olive oil, Cajun seasoning, cayenne pepper, and Worcestershire sauce in a small bowl. Place zucchinis, onions, yellow squash in a bowl and cover with the olive oil mixture. Salt to taste.

2. Cover bowl, then marinate vegetables in the refrigerator for at least 30 minutes. Warm an outdoor

grill for high heat and lightly oil grate. Place marinated vegetable pieces on skewers or directly on the grill. Cook 5 minutes until done.

Nutrition:

Calories: 95

Fat: 7g

Carbs: 8g

Protein: 2g

87. Purple Potatoes with Onions, Mushrooms, and Capers

Preparation Time: 10 minutes

Cooking Time: 25 minutes

Servings: 4

Ingredients:

- 6 purple potatoes, scrubbed

- 3 tbsp. extra virgin olive oil

- 1 large red onion, chopped

- 8 oz. fresh mushrooms, sliced

- Salt and pepper to taste

- ¼ tsp chili pepper flakes

- 1 tbsp. capers, drained and chopped

- 1 tsp fresh tarragon, chopped

Directions:

1. Slice each potato into wedges. Heat your skillet over medium heat, then put 1 tbsp of olive oil.

2. Cook the onion plus mushrooms within 5 minutes.

3. Transfer it into a bowl and set aside. Heat 2 more tbsp of olive oil on high heat in the same skillet and add the potato wedges.

4. Flavor it with salt plus pepper, and allow to cook within 10 minutes.

5. Adjust the heat to medium, sprinkle the potato wedges with red pepper flakes, and allow to cook within 10 more minutes. Mix in the onion plus mushroom mixture, toss the vegetables together and mix in the capers and fresh tarragon.

Nutrition:

Calories: 215

Fat: 6g

Carbs: 23g

Protein: 3g

88. Vegetarian Stuffed Peppers

Preparation Time: 10 minutes

Cooking Time: 70 minutes

Servings: 6

Ingredients:

- 1 ½ cups brown rice, uncooked
- 6 large green bell peppers
- 3 tbsp. soy sauce
- 3 tbsp. dry red wine
- 1 tsp vegetarian Worcestershire sauce
- 1 ½ cups extra firm tofu
- 1/2 cup sweetened dried cranberries
- ¼ cup walnuts, chopped
- ½ cup Parmesan, grated
- Salt and pepper, to taste
- 2 cups tomato sauce
- 2 tbsp. brown sugar

Directions:

1. Preheat oven to 350°F. Boil 3 cups water in a saucepan, then mix in the rice. Lower the heat, cover, and simmer within 40 minutes. Meanwhile, core and green seed peppers, leaving bottoms intact.

2. Place peppers in a microwavable dish with about ½" of water in the bottom. Microwave on high for 6 minutes.

3. In a small saucepan, bring soy sauce, wine, and Worcestershire sauce to a simmer. Add tofu and simmer until the liquid is absorbed.

4. Combine rice, tofu, cranberries, nuts, cheese, salt, and pepper in a large bowl and mix well — Pack rice firmly into peppers.

5. Return peppers to the dish you first microwaved them in and baked for 25 to 30 minutes, or until lightly browned on top.

6. Meanwhile, mix tomato sauce and brown sugar in a small saucepan over low heat. Heat until hot. Serve stuffed peppers with the tomato sauce spooned over each serving.

Nutrition:

Calories: 250

Carbs: 22g

Fat: 10g

Protein: 17g

Conclusion

Congratulations! You now know how to follow the Sirtfood diet diligently and lose weight healthily and consistently.

There are several diets out there. Dieting has become an industry of its own, with videos, books, blogs, and all sorts of diet pills, supplements, and other items accessible to customers. At the same time, Western nations are becoming more health-conscious and overweight, and, as a result, there is a rising demand for information on diets and items related to weight loss. However, what's not much of it is solid, useful information about how to successfully diet-that is, how to effectively lose weight and keep it off.

Anyone can lose weight by following one of the many fad diets available. Still, these diets have a few fatal flaws. They generally do not provide you with a nutritionally healthy diet; they're not intended for anything other than short-term weight loss and, perhaps worst of all, they generally do not provide you with any sleep.

However, you don't need fad diet plans or diet pills to eat effectively; you need the right details on what to do and what to avoid when you're trying to lose weight. The SirtFood diet is 70-80 percent raw and also contains the following:

Motivation: If you are not motivated to lose weight and improve your health, you probably won't be successful regardless of what kind of diet you follow. It needs the self-discipline to avoid food mistakes, and to get enough exercise, you need to lose weight and keep it off. Without that, nothing is going to work for you in the long run.

Water: Drinking plenty of water is something you can do in the first place because it is so crucial to good health. Drinking eight or more cups of water a day helps your digestive system work more efficiently, helping you lose weight, and drinking water also helps you feel full; in many cases, you may be thirsty when you feel hungry. Drink a glass of water when you're feeling hungry and make a point of getting a glass before meals; you might be shocked by how much less you consume by mealtimes.

Daily Drill: We all know that we need regular exercise, especially if we're trying to lose weight. If you're not getting some form of exercise regularly, try starting small with a half-hour walk every day and work your way up to more intensive exercise and longer workouts. Usually, you'll get the best results with half an hour to 45 minutes of exercise at least three or four days a week. Even if you don't have a lot of spare time on your day, try to put in a little physical exercise whenever you can, take the stairs instead of the elevator, walk to the store instead of driving, or to take a cab, and so on – every little bit helps you lose excess weight and keep it off.

Good, Nutritionally Balanced Diets: We all have an excellent idea of what we should eat; fresh vegetables and fruit, whole grains, small amounts of healthy fats like olive oil, fish, and other lean meats. It is more important to keep your mind clear: refined flours, sugar, processed foods, and any food or beverage filled with preservatives and other artificial ingredients. Get into the habit of carefully reading food labels and, if possible, cook your food with fresh ingredients instead of purchasing pre-made packaged food. It's OK to get a little out of your diet once in a while. But most of the time, you need to stick to the plan.

When you get used to eating healthy, you will find that you quickly lose your appetite for less nutritious choices, and, combined with daily exercise, it will make it easier to stay away from the weight you've gained.

I hope this cookbook will help you reach your wellness and weight loss goals naturally.

I love you

With love Vilma J. Hernandez

Lightning Source UK Ltd.
Milton Keynes UK
UKHW020234220521
384136UK00001B/5